# EVERY WOMAN'S GUIDE to ANTI-AGING MEDICINE

Eric S. Berger, M.D.

Every Woman's Guide to Anti-Aging Medicine

Copyright © 2012 by Eric S. Berger, M.D.

All rights reserved.

No part of this book may be reproduced or transmitted in any form without the express written permission of the author.

The information contained in this book is intended for educational purposes only. The author is not rendering professional advice or services to the individual reader.

ISBN-13: 978-1477584385

To order additional copies, please visit:

www.amazon.com

## ABOUT THE AUTHOR

Dr. Eric Berger completed specialty training in Ear Nose & Throat/Head & Neck Surgery at the Albert Einstein College of Medicine--Montefiore Medical Center in New York City. He did a fellowship in Facial Cosmetic Surgery at Graduate Hospital in Philadelphia. He founded a successful practice in Washington State and was elected Chairman of the Department of Surgery at Grays Harbor Hospital in 1986.

He returned to New York as Medical Director of the American Council on Science and Health, an educational organization dedicated to public health, nutrition, and cutting-edge scientific issues.

Dr. Berger is a Board Certified Fellow of the American Academy of Anti-Aging Medicine. He is specially certified in the laser cosmetic procedures; teaches laser technique to physicians and aestheticians; and is a member of the American Society for Laser Medicine and Surgery.

In addition to writing, Dr. Berger is also a film maker, and bi-lingual in English and Spanish.

## Dedication

To my father, Irving, who loved science and logic, and knew a thousand jokes. His irreverent sense of humor surfaces in everything I do, say and write.

To my mother, Sylvia, who was too smart by half. She relished the English language and taught me by example the power of unbridled sarcasm.

I wish you were here to read this book. I think you'd like it.

**Special Acknowledgment**

To Sam Abady; brilliant lawyer, masterful editor and faithful friend. This book could not have been written without your invaluable editorial input.

To Dr. Jane Watson whose keen medical insights and invaluable research added greatly to this book.

To Gerard & Regan Connolly; your encouragement, friendship and love have motivated and inspired me for twenty six years.

## Contents

**ABOUT THE AUTHOR** .................................................................. 3
Dedication ................................................................................. 5
Special Acknowledgment ........................................................... 7
Prologue: Aging is a Disease ................................................... 13
**Introduction: What is Anti-Aging Medicine?** ...................... 15
**Chapter 1: The Skin You're In** ............................................. 17
Cellular Slowdown .................................................................. 19
The Epidermis ........................................................................ 19
The Dermis ............................................................................. 24
Other Dermal Denizens .......................................................... 27
Skin Toxins -- Cigarettes & Exhaust Fumes .......................... 30
Carbon Monoxide ................................................................... 31
Free Radicals ......................................................................... 31
Sunshine is Not Your Friend .................................................. 34
Suffocating Skin ..................................................................... 36
Recap ..................................................................................... 39
**Chapter 2: Saving Your Skin** ............................................... 41
The Myth of Fancy Soap ........................................................ 41
The Acid Mantle ..................................................................... 44
How Bad is Your Acne? .......................................................... 45
Facials and Exfoliation ........................................................... 48
Moisturizers ............................................................................ 49
Sun Protection Factor ............................................................ 51
Recap ..................................................................................... 53

**Chapter 3: "If you keep making that face..."** ............... **55**
BOTOX® at 30? ................................................................. 55
Fillers Fill. That's All They Do ........................................... 59
Juvederm® ....................................................................... 61
Radiesse® and the "Liquid Face Lift" ............................... 64
Recap ............................................................................... 66
**Chapter 4: The Light Fantastic** ................................... **67**
Photo-Thermo-Lysis ......................................................... 67
Tightening and Resurfacing the Skin with Light ............... 70
Spot Treatment ................................................................ 76
Lasers and People of Color ............................................. 77
Recap ............................................................................... 80
**Chapter 5: Hormonal High Jinks** ................................ **83**
Estrogen ........................................................................... 85
The Downside of Estrogen - Breast Disease and Blood Clots ....... 90
Progesterone .................................................................... 91
Recap ............................................................................... 94
**Chapter 6: Sea Salt and Endless Fatigue** ................. **97**
Thyroid Hormone .............................................................. 97
Recap ............................................................................. 102
**Chapter 7: You're Stressing Me Out!** ...................... **105**
Chronic Fatigue .............................................................. 105
Adrenalin and Cortisol ................................................... 106
Eight Vital Hours ............................................................ 109
Sleep vs. Hormones ...................................................... 110
Sleep and Stay Thin ...................................................... 110
Sleep Refreshes Skin .................................................... 111

The Dracula Hormone .................................................................. 111
Recap ............................................................................................ 113
**Chapter 8: When Does Growth Stop? ...................................... 117**
The Master Hormone ..................................................................... 118
Measuring HGH via IGF-1 ............................................................. 119
Side Effects ................................................................................... 121
HGH Secretagogues ..................................................................... 123
Recap ............................................................................................ 124
**Chapter 9: She Broke Her Hip and Fell Down ........................ 127**
Osteoporosis ................................................................................. 127
Finding and Fixing Weak Bones ................................................... 133
Diet Tips ........................................................................................ 134
Recap ............................................................................................ 135
**Chapter 10: The Body Extreme ................................................ 137**
Prehistoric You .............................................................................. 141
Kick Start Your Diet ....................................................................... 146
All Sugar Is Not Created Equal ..................................................... 149
Exercise is Essential ..................................................................... 152
Bikram Yoga .................................................................................. 160
Vitamins and Minerals on the Cheap ........................................... 161
Recap ............................................................................................ 165
**Chapter 11: Cosmetic Surgery ................................................. 167**
The Eyes Have It ........................................................................... 168
Nobody Nose ................................................................................. 170
Abreast of the Latest Developments ............................................ 172
Recap ............................................................................................ 175

**Chapter 12: Longevity Myths and Facts** ...................................**177**
Fitting Into Your Genes ................................................................178
Fat Is Definitely Out. Is Thin Really In? ........................................179
Child Bearing and Longevity .......................................................181
Recap ..........................................................................................183
**Chapter 13: The Future of Anti-Aging Medicine** .....................**185**
A Lesson in History .....................................................................186
Embryonic Stem Cells.................................................................188
Telomeres and Anti-Telomerase .................................................190
Anti-Aging Physicians .................................................................191

## Prologue: Aging is a Disease

The Merriam-Webster online dictionary defines "disease" as:

*"A condition of the living animal body, or of one of its parts that impairs normal functioning and is typically manifested by distinguishing signs and symptoms."*

It's important to recognize that the words "bacteria," "viruses" and "tumors" are not part of the definition. Certainly, no one can deny these things cause a significant number of diseases, but we often overlook one of the most powerful disease-causing entities: time.

Yup, Time.

From the first tick of the clock at the moment of your birth you begin an uphill swing toward becoming a healthy adult. This happens at around ages 16-20. Then you reach a biological plateau when everything levels off for a while.

Barring unforeseen events (bacteria, viruses, and tumors for example), your physical health is pretty much stable until age 40-45. In a perfect world, your hormone levels, hair texture, hair distribution, skin condition and metabolism have remained stable until you start to reach menopause.

But what, exactly, is the "perfect world"?

From your body's perspective, it means a world with an undamaged ozone layer to protect you from ultraviolet (UV) radiation; there are no cars, buses and factories spewing pollutants into the pristine air; meat and poultry are savory and pure, produced without chemical additives like hormones and antibiotics; and life is an endless stream of stress free, 72° F, cloudless, joy-filled days.

This world may have once existed but, if it did, we were cast out after Eve ate the apple. (And they tell us, "An apple a day keeps the doctor away.")

In the *real world* -- our world – UV radiation, pollutants and a million other factors ravage and destroy your delicate body from the moment you start your life journey.

Fortunately, until you reach adulthood, the growth process itself protects you from the most serious dangers. Once you have traveled the road to adulthood - once growth stops and everything levels off - you're on your own against the elements.

When growth stops is when Anti-Aging Medicine becomes vitally important. It's a relatively new specialty, practiced by physicians who know that the correct regimen of diet, supplementation, exercise and hormones can change old age into truly "Golden Years."

Eric S. Berger, M.D.

## Introduction: What is Anti-Aging Medicine?

Many people erroneously view anti-aging medicine as a synonym for skin care. The advertising and fashion worlds pitch skin care products to women ages of 40-60, the demographic group which most frequently purchases products for tired, spotted and wrinkled skin.

There is certainly no lack of medical resources explaining the basic function of skin, how it ages, popular laser treatments, essential maintenance by licensed aestheticians and the use of BOTOX® and fillers. (I'm frequently surprised by the confusion that exists between these two common, yet totally different, injection treatments.)

The problem is, many of these resources are biased and exist only to promote a particular line of products or treatments developed by a particular physician.

In reviewing this literature, one is struck by two important facts:

- first, while there are many anti-aging skin care books in print, few address *complete* anti-aging medicine for women; and

- second, women (and men) learn basic healthcare habits like tooth brushing early in life, and these habits continue essentially unchanged into adulthood and later life. The biggest difference between the sexes is that men tend to ignore health matters and wait until things to go wrong, while women are more conscientious about routine maintenance.

This book is different. It provides a succinct but comprehensive overview of Anti-Aging Medicine for women 15-90, and covers the entire female body, not just the skin. Within these pages I explain anti-aging skin care; hormone replacement therapy; diet and supplements; and exercise; all in an accessible, understandable way.

I can't promise you a longer life. You can follow every suggestion and still succumb to an undiagnosed genetic disorder, viral epidemic or traffic accident. But absent these unpredictable events, if you follow my guidelines you can live wonderful, miraculous years beyond what you ever expected.

## Chapter 1: The Skin You're In

Most people are surprised to learn that skin is an organ, and as just don't seem to take skin seriously. They fail to appreciate that skin has a vital biological function and purpose. So much attention is devoted to skin *appearance* that virtually no attention is devoted to skin *health*.

In reality, every physician and skin care specialist should know (and teach you) that these two aspects are indivisible. Healthy skin is attractive, glowing and wrinkle-free, while unhealthy skin is unattractive, dry and furrowed.

In fact, many elements which cause skin to age also cause aging in the rest of the body. That makes the skin is an excellent starting point to explain general concepts of anti-aging.

The general thought behind modern skin care is directed towards taking women age sixty and trying to make them look fifty, or women age fifty and trying to make them look forty. Strenuous efforts are dedicated to separate vulnerable women from their money by pushing highly overpriced cosmeceuticals and potions, and practically coercing women to endure unnecessary or ineffective treatments.

Anyone who watches television on any channel at any hour of the day or night cannot help but notice the enormous increase in advertisements for "anti-aging" skin care products. These products all have one thing in common: they promise to turn back the clock.

One ad which I find particularly offensive ends with a voiceover proclaiming their product "can make you look ten years younger!" The lovely young actress then smiles seductively into the camera and says, "Ten years. I'll take that!"

The paradigm of removing existing signs of age should be called *Un-Aging Medicine*. It represents expensive, complicated, and often harmful attempts to turn back the clock.

Sadly, it never really works as well as *slowing* the aging process before it starts to ravage your skin and your body. The results of trying to turn back the clock don't begin to approximate the look of youthful skin. Rather, women who use these products look like women with old skin in a state of desperation.

Don't get me wrong. I am not saying that, after a certain age, there is no hope of skin rejuvenation. But it's time to throw some realistic goals into the mix. Certainly, lasers and facials, well chosen products, BOTOX® and fillers nearly always can improve the appearance of women at any age. In addition, recent technological and chemical advances make it possible to restore at least partial health to severely damaged skin. But intervening after the fact pales in effectiveness to what can be accomplished if skin care begins early, before the damage is done.

To see the big picture, it is necessary to understand how skin works and all the reasons it gets old, thin, wrinkled and dry. There are environmental, lifestyle and illness-driven aspects of aging skin.

## Cellular Slowdown
Skin is fascinating stuff. Under the right circumstances, it not only looks great, but serves a multitude of essential purposes. It is thin, tough and resilient, and does a great job of healing itself.

## The Epidermis
For starters, skin is your protector. It keeps the outside out and the inside in. Without your skin, all the moisture in your body would evaporate in a matter of hours, while bacteria and other external infectious agents would quickly move inside. Your skin's protective surface is called the Epidermis, the outermost layer. One of the most surprising things about the Epidermis is that it is only about $1/16^{th}$ of an inch thick.

There are four important sub-layers of Epidermis, but it is easier to think of it as one, ever-changing layer because each layer derives from just one kind of cell, the Basal Cells. These cells change shape, size and content to become, in turn, Spiny, Granular and, finally, Horny Cells. (Stop giggling. This is serious stuff.)

Think of epidermal basal cells like a field of magic balloons, each one filled with a watery gel. Every balloon has the amazing ability to divide into two balloons which are identical in every way, and each of those then divides into two more balloons, and so on. Even as the number of cells grows, the layer stays the same size, because, as new balloons are created the older balloons are pushed upwards. A diagram makes this clear.

The lowest layer is what we commonly refer to as the Basal Layer (in Latin, *Stratum Basale or "layer" and "base"*). The Basal Layer is the *only* layer of the Epidermis which can divide and reproduce its cells.

As the older Basal Cells are pushed upward, they begin to transform. First, some of their water is lost, which causes the gel inside to thicken.

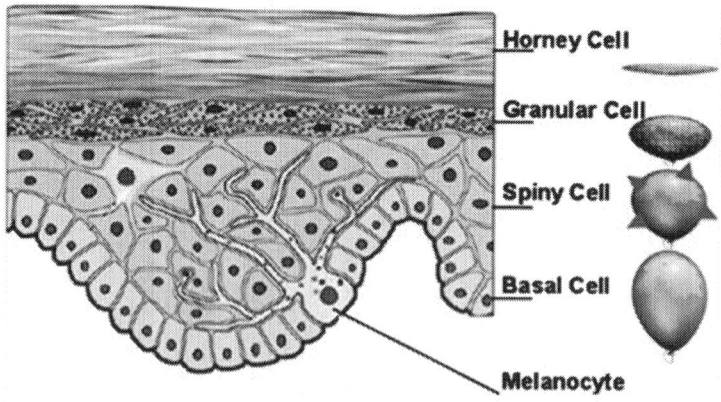

Then the surfaces of the individual balloons start to stick together. The outer cell wall develops actual spines which make them stick together even better, and explains why we call this layer the Spinous or Spiny Layer (*Stratum Spinosum*).

Because the Spiny balloons are denser and tightly stuck together, this is the layer most resistant to mechanical injury. When you slip on your four-inch heels and land on cobblestones, or lose your grip while peeling, slicing and dicing your Whole Foods organic salad, it is the Spiny Layer which protects you from cuts and abrasions.

The Base balloons keep dividing and pushing each other upward so that, eventually, the older Spiny Balloons get pushed upward, too. As they rise, Spiny Balloons lose even more water, and the interior gel becomes very dry and granular. The cell wall also begins to form a hard, armor-like substance called Keratin. Keratin is a very tough protein also found in hair, animal hooves, and horns.

The cells of this layer are filled with granular material of dried gel, so this layer is called the Granular Layer (*Stratum Granulosum*).

As the upward push of Basal Cells continues, the Granular balloons go through their final structural change. The last of the gel granules disappears, and the dry, flakey, stuck-together cells are just like plates of hard, Keratin armor. Usually about 10-14 layers of these Keratin plates cover and protect the skin. Because Keratin is a key component of animal horn, this is called the Horny Layer (*Stratum Corneum*).

When we are young, this constant process of Basal Cells becoming Spiny Cells, Granular Cells and finally, Horny

Cells, is quite rapid. As teenagers, we turn over a fresh layer of skin cells every 7-10 days. That's why young skin glows and has that fresh, rosy appearance.

As we age, however, the Basal Cells get tired and start to wear out. They no longer have the hormones, blood flow and metabolism to multiply and divide as frequently as they did when we were young. They've been damaged and injured by a million physical and chemical insults. As a result, by age thirty, the epidermal turnover process takes about thirty days instead of seven. At age 60, full skin turnover takes about sixty days. That means that for two months you're wearing the same old flakey, dry skin.

As production of new cells slows down with age, a larger number of our epidermal cells are the flat, dry, flaky keratin-filled plates. That's one of the reasons our skin becomes thinner and more fragile as we get older.

Remember that those 10-14 layers of keratin armor plates when you consider splurging on expensive skin treatments and moisturizers. "Magic ingredients" in that $300 a jar moisturizer simply cannot get past those 14 keratin cell layers and into your deeper granular or spiny cell layers, so using expensive moisturizers is a colossal waste of money. Practically none of whatever you apply is actually absorbed, and most of it is simply washed down the drain.

The Basal Layer also contains a small number of two other types of cells: Melanocytes and Undifferentiated Cells.

Melanocytes produce the brown pigment Melanin. Melanin is the stuff that makes People of Color colorful. Melanocytes react to sunlight. The quest to increase Melanin production is what inspires people *without* color to lie in the sun for hours so they can look more like People of Color.

Interestingly, blacks, whites and Latinos have about the same number of Melanocytes, but the amount and structure of the melanin produced by them is different.

Excessive sun can cause skin cancers, and melanin is an amazing sun-blocker, which explains why two skin cancers, Basal Cell Carcinoma and Melanoma, are rare in People of Color. Nature gave them a highly effective natural SPF (Sun Protection Factor) in their skin.

Like the other cells in the Basal Layer, Undifferentiated Cells can reproduce and are particularly vulnerable during the reproduction process (aren't we all). This means that exposure to UV radiation can cause the DNA in these cells to mutate and change into cancerous cells.

Undifferentiated Cells were recently identified as the cells which cause Basal Cell Carcinoma, the most common skin cancer, rather than the Basal Cells themselves as previously thought. At some point, medicine may change the name of this skin cancer from Basal Cell Carcinoma to Undifferentiated Cell Carcinoma.

## The Dermis

It's important to remember that, despite being composed of several layers, the Epidermis is only about 1/16$^{th}$ of an inch thick. If your skin were composed solely of the Epidermis, it would hang on you like wet paper towels -- a loose, formless, easily torn sheet.

Fortunately, beneath the Epidermis lies the Dermis which provides scaffolding - a framework of form, flexibility and strength to support the weaker, thinner Epidermis.

The Dermis is about two to three times as thick as the Epidermis; about 1/8$^{th}$ of an inch thick in most areas, and is many times stronger than the Epidermis. Its strength comes from its structure. The Dermis contains specialized cells called Fibroblasts, fiber producing cells which, as the name indicates, produce fibers. These fibers are predominantly of two types: Collagen and Elastin.

Elastin gives the skin elasticity and flexibility; it makes skin stretchy. However, the role of Elastin is not as important as Collagen in the overall appearance of skin.

Collagen is produced in strands which form a thick, dense, flexible mesh or matrix within the Dermis. Under a microscope, the appearance of the collagen matrix is similar in appearance to the matrix of wood fibers found in ordinary paper.

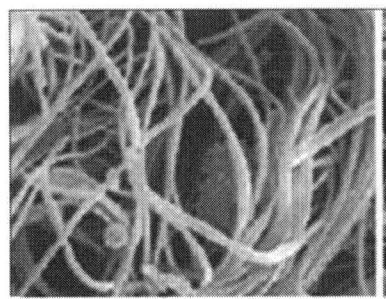 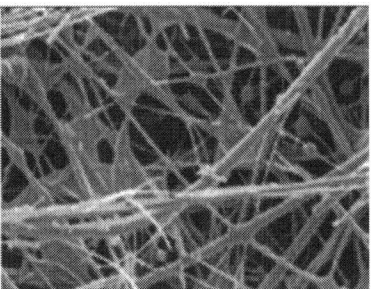

**Dermal Collagen Matrix**     **Paper Fiber Matrix**

When the collagen matrix is smooth, the surface of the skin is smooth. However, when we make facial expressions, facial muscles crumple the collagen matrix causing it to wrinkle just like paper. If we wrinkle it repeatedly the wrinkles turn into permanent creases, also known as furrows.

The wrinkling process begins early. Many women already develop slight furrows where their facial expressions are most active in their early twenties. Fortunately, young people produce an abundance of new collagen fibers which constantly repair the ongoing damage.

As we age, fibroblast function slows down, which results in collagen production slowing down, too.

At that point, we've repeated the wrinkling and bending process millions of times and *active wrinkles,* only visible during facial movement like smiling, became *passive wrinkles* or furrows which are visible all the time. As we age, permanent creases appear more frequently and are more resistant to repair.

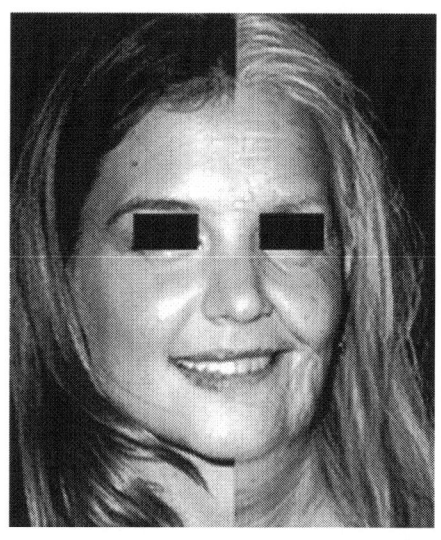

The Dermis has two distinct layers. The upper layer where the Epidermis and Dermis meet is called the Papillary Layer. Papillae (plural for Papilla) are tiny bumps all over the surface of the Dermis. These bumps cause the surface area where the Epidermis and Dermis meet to be much larger than with a flat surface union without the bumps.

This large surface area is important because the Epidermis has no blood supply of its own. Every drop of moisture, nourishment and sustenance in the Epidermis is passed to it from the Dermis through the blood vessels in the Papillary Layer.

The fine, shallow wrinkles in the faces of old people are proof that collagen production slows down as we age. The Papillary Layer of the Dermis changes from a smooth, flowing surface into an endless sea of tiny, dry grooves.

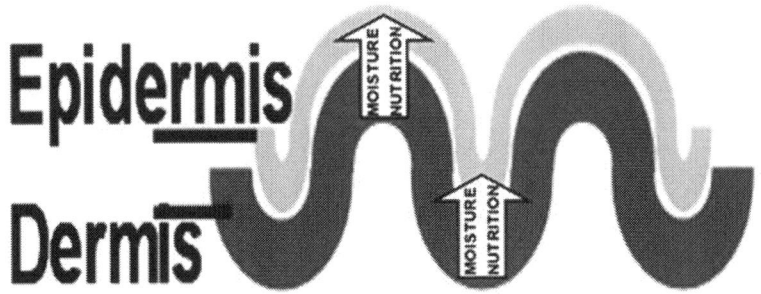

The second layer of collagen is deeper, denser and stronger. It is called the Reticular Collagen Layer, and that is where deeper facial furrows form. The constant folding and bending of the Reticular Layer and corresponding slowdown in collagen production are primarily responsible for the furrowing process.

## Other Dermal Denizens

The Dermis is home to a few other important structures. Among these are hair follicles, oil (sebaceous) glands, scent glands and sweat glands.

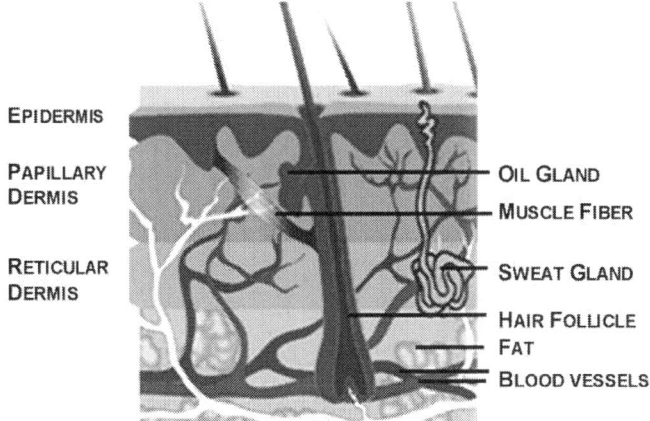

To Propionibacteria Acnes or *p. acnes,* the bacteria responsible for causing acne, the sebum produced by oil glands is a wonderful delicacy.

Bacteria are living microorganisms, and like all other living organisms, bacteria eat and excrete. What they eat is sebum and what they excrete is Porphyrin (pronounced por-fer-in). The simplest definition of the type of porphyrin in your pores is "bacterial poop." The pores of unclean skin are filled with bacterial poop. It clogs pores, exposes us to chronic skin irritation, and feeds acne.

Porphyrin is also extremely corrosive. It destroys collagen walls of the pores and therefore enlarges the pores. Almost everyone needs to learn to cleanse his or her face more carefully and thoroughly, especially on and around the nose. It's important to scrub deep into the grooves behind the nostrils. Failure to adequately wash these areas is one important reason they so often become the site of acne breakouts and the first areas to develop gaping pores as we age.

The good news is that porphyrins are fairly easy to remove with careful washing, especially if the layers of dead surface cells blocking pore openings have been removed by exfoliation and microdermabrasion.

The importance of monthly, professional deep facials and exfoliations cannot be overemphasized.

The next Dermal structure, the Sweat Glands, cool the body. Sweating covers our skin surface with moisture which evaporates, and surface evaporation is a natural air conditioning system. To illustrate the point, wear a dampened tee shirt and stand in front of a fan. The air flow will cause water to evaporate and you'll feel cold.

Tiny veins and capillaries dilate during periods of heat exposure, too. Blood vessel expansion brings more of our blood supply to the skin and allows more heat to dissipate from the body surface.

Both sweat and scent gland secretions contain pheromones (pronounced fer-o-mones). These are the subtle, natural scents animals secrete to stimulate attraction and mating activity in many species. A male moth can detect the scent of a female moth despite miles of separation. He can follow that scent directly to its source by flying in the direction of the increasing concentration of pheromones in the air.

The role of pheromones in human sexual attraction is a hotly debated scientific topic. Ongoing studies have yet to identify a specific human attraction pheromone, but science is getting close. The economic incentive for this research is obvious. Isolate and reproduce a human sex pheromone and you will have created an authentic "love potion."

If this happens, synthetic perfumes and after shaves will immediately become obsolete. We will attract mates by spraying ourselves with bio-identical human pheromones developed by studying the chemical composition of human sweat and the secretions of scent glands.

If you're one of those wet blankets who mutters, "Get a room!" when you cross paths with an amorous couple locked in a public display of affection, be prepared to spend a lot more time at home. A working pheromone spray will render us all practically irresistible to one another.

## Skin Toxins -- Cigarettes & Exhaust Fumes

Let's revisit an important fact I mentioned earlier: the Epidermis has no blood supply of its own. All the tiny arteries and capillaries that feed the Epidermis run through the Dermis and the fat pad below it.

Therefore, it's logical to assume that anything which impedes blood flow and the blood's ability to carry oxygen to the cells will be very harmful to the skin.

Here are two simple equations:

No blood supply & oxygen = No epidermal turnover = Dry, irritated flaky skin

No blood supply & oxygen = No collagen production = Saggy, wrinkled, loose skin

*There is nothing more dangerous to small vessel blood flow, cell oxygenation and your overall health than cigarettes.*

If you want beautiful, smooth, healthy skin for the rest of your life, don't smoke – ever – period. If you smoke, quit. Smoking is absolutely the worst thing for your skin (and the lungs, heart, arteries and veins).

Smoking destroys the lining in blood vessels which, in the skin, are quite small anyway, and makes these vessels highly susceptible to blockage.

## Carbon Monoxide

Slow burning, packed tobacco does not burn completely; a significant portion of every puff is Carbon Monoxide (CO as opposed to $CO_2$). This is the same stuff which spews out of your car's exhaust pipe. Carbon Monoxide is the poisonous gas people intent on committing suicide breathe while they try to kill themselves, sitting in a closed garage with the car running.

How does carbon monoxide cause injury and death? Our cells require oxygen to live. Red blood cells carry oxygen to the tissues. Think of red blood cells as seats on a train and oxygen and carbon monoxide molecules as potential passengers competing for those seats.

Carbon monoxide molecules get preferential seating. Carbon monoxide binds with red blood cells *permanently*, thus preventing oxygen from ever reaching your skin. Carbon monoxide literally causes your skin cells (all your cells, in fact) to suffocate from oxygen deprivation.

## Free Radicals

If blocking oxygen from getting to your cells weren't bad enough, both cigarettes and exhaust fumes contain large amounts of Free Radicals. In basic chemistry we learn that every atom has a nucleus at the center, and electrons which orbit around it. Atoms look like tiny solar systems. The number of electrons determines how one atom reacts with other atoms. Every electron must be accounted for in every chemical reaction. For example, if one atom has four electrons and another atom has three electrons, when they join properly they will have a total of seven electrons.

In the most basic sense, Free Radicals are *electron thieves*. Free Radicals are electron deplete compounds with fewer electrons than required to keep them stable. Think of them as *electron disabled* (no doubt, some will insist that description is politically incorrect. Shall I call them "electron challenged", instead?)

To remedy their electron deficiency, Free Radicals steal electrons from any nearby healthy atoms, forcing the victimized atoms to rob other atoms, and so on, leading to an endless chain reaction of electron robberies.

During this cascade of electron robberies, important molecules like the DNA in our skin cells become very vulnerable to mutation. These mutations can interrupt the formation of healthy collagen, cause the production of abnormal Basal Cells and Undifferentiated Cells, and can lead to skin cancer.

Let's face it, you can't stop breathing, and you probably won't move to the countryside just to avoid exhaust fumes. But you can stop smoking. Inhaling even a few cigarettes a day is like crawling behind a slow moving car and deliberately inhaling its exhaust. Not a pretty picture.

Every Woman's Guide to Anti-Aging Medicine

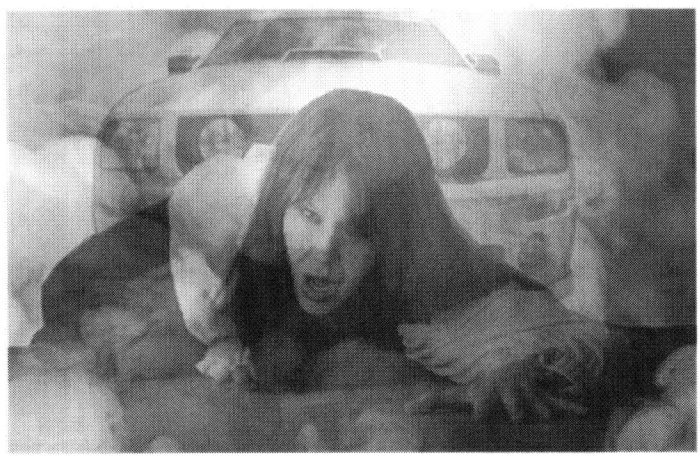

Most young smokers start smoking for social reasons. They think smoking makes them look cool. Young people believe they are addiction- proof and never expect they'll get hooked on nicotine.

Gram for gram, nicotine is as addictive as crack cocaine. In a very real sense, tobacco company executives are no different than your average neighborhood crack dealers, except they work in office buildings wearing suits and ties, instead of on street corners wearing tee shirts and jeans.

You might be saying to yourself, "I've heard this sermon a million times." And you're right. Yet, tragically, *most new smokers are young women between the ages of 16 and 25*, so I don't really care if I'm being repetitive.

What makes matters worse is that many of these young women also take birth control pills. Recent university studies conclusively prove that women increase the risk of having first-time heart attacks or strokes by thirty times -- that's

3000% -- when they smoke twenty-five cigarettes or more a day and take a daily, low-dose birth control pill.

Have I made my point?

## Sunshine is Not Your Friend

A young patient recently told me she lies out in the sun to "make Vitamin D." That's a pretty lame excuse. First of all, she was Caucasian and Caucasians only needs between 10-20 minutes *a week* of direct sunlight to create more than enough Vitamin D.

African Americans need between 30-50 minutes a week because the extra Melanin in their skin is such an effective sunscreen.

Further, taking a daily multi-vitamin supplement with Vitamin D is more than sufficient to avoid the need for prolonged sun exposure at all. If you don't like taking pills, Vitamin D is found in tuna and salmon as well as in fortified foods like milk and breakfast cereals.

Why is this important? Once upon a time, somewhere between the start of the industrial revolution and the ban on aerosol spray cans containing chlorofluorocarbons (CFCs), the earth had an undamaged atmospheric shield called the Ozone Layer. UV light was reflected off of the Ozone Layer, thus protecting us by preventing too much of the sun's UV light from reaching both the earth's surface and our skin.

UV light in excess is extremely harmful. It causes sunburn, Basal Cell carcinoma (*the* most common of all cancers), cataracts and direct DNA damage to the cells which makes them mutate and become cancerous.

In 1974, scientists discovered that certain aerosol propellants containing CFCs were destroying the Ozone Layer. In 1976, Congress passed the Toxic Substances Control Act which banned these substances in manufacturing, but internationally, they were not banned until 1989 when 196 nations entered a multi-lateral treaty called The Montreal Protocol on Substances That Deplete the Ozone Layer.

It's disgraceful that it took fifteen years for the world community to finally act. (It frequently takes too long for scientific discoveries to translate into governmental regulations. We still have not limited tanning parlors or the sale of personal UV sun lamps, even though science definitively proved tanning beds and sun lamps cause skin cancer.)

We are constantly bombarded by intense UV radiation. To make matters worse, many of us are still convinced that being tan makes us more attractive.

Maybe it does, but there are new and improved self-tanners which do not require overexposure to harmful UV radiation. In the early days of artificial tanning lotions, you'd get a orange instead of tan, and look like a giant tomato. Happily, most modern self-tanners actually make you look naturally golden tan. One of the best self-tanners on the market is

Clarins. For a very reasonable price, it provides a rich, golden tan without giving you cancer.

By now you might be thinking, "Why is this particular subject so important to Dr. Berger?" OK. It's time to share a story from my own life. During summers in high school, I worked as a lifeguard. This was a few years before UV light and cancer were linked. Six days a week, I sat in the sun, whistle around my neck and slathered in baby oil and Iodine on an imposing, ten-foot high lifeguard's chair from 10:00 A.M. when the pool opened until 8:00 P.M. when it closed. No protective chair umbrella, no sunscreen. In fact, in those days, sunscreen didn't even exist. I thought I looked pretty cool up on that chair with white Zinc Oxide ointment on my nose.

A colleague diagnosed my first Basal Cell skin cancer about *thirty years later*. The time between UV exposure and actual cancer can be quite long. I've had over a dozen cancerous patches removed since then. My dermatologist jokes that, if he keeps cutting little pieces off of me, they'll be able to bury me in a matchbox. That's funny, but I'm not ROTF or LMAO. It is important that this doesn't happen to you. First and foremost, remember that excessive sun exposure is dangerous.

## Suffocating Skin
Makeup is a dirty word. Makeup suffocates the skin.

Unless you have unsightly blemishes, pigmented spots or a grapevine scar from a sword fight, I guarantee you will look sexier without a painted face; cleaner, fresher and more approachable.

Most men with taste prefer women naked -- no makeup whatsoever. After a few hours, even the best makeup gets sticky because natural sebaceous oils constantly produced by your skin, co-mingled with sweat, increases the surface adhesion of all makeup.

And there is nothing worse for your skin than going to sleep in your makeup.

Here's an interesting scenario for you to consider: It's Friday morning. You traveled to work through dusty city streets and air filled with vehicle exhaust, allergenic pollens, construction dust and hundreds of other more disgusting pollutants. You sat at your desk all day as invisible smog, traveling through office ductwork and air vents, was deposited on your skin. [The FDA reports that indoor office air is often more dangerous than outdoor air.]

Later that evening, you joined your BFF for dinner and an evening of clubbing.

You held your breath as you entered and left the club to avoid inhaling the haze of tobacco smoke created by smokers gathered around the entrance who, in a truly civilized society, would be compelled to puff far from the doorway. The smoke did, however, manage to stick to your makeup, sebaceous oil and sweat.

Finally, you met "that guy." He bought you a few drinks, chatted you up, and next thing you know, you're back at his place. God only knows, you can't let him see you without makeup in the morning, so you just leave it on – with the skin oil, sweat, smog, cigarette smoke, and other environmental pollutants that settled on your skin since you arose that morning.

The smog and smoke contain plenty of the Free Radicals. Every minute of that romantic night you were destroying collagen, widening your pores and wrinkling your precious skin which lies buried beneath that horrendous mixture of makeup, oil, sweat, cigarette smoke and pollutants.

Ask any male friend with his olfactory sense intact. He'll confirm the makeup, left on overnight, smells.

Ah, romance!

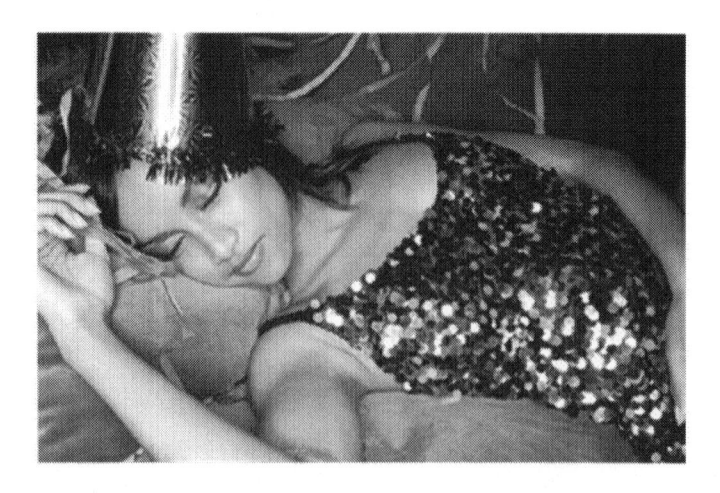

The solution to this dilemma is simple. Carry a "skin kit" containing small bottles of your favorite cleanser, night cream and eye serum in a plastic bag in your purse. Better yet, you could just bite the bullet, throw away the majority of your makeup, and start going naked.

## Recap

- Our skin is a vital organ designed, among other things, to keep the inside in and the outside out, regulate body temperature and prevent infections.

- As we age, all aspects of skin structure deteriorate, especially cell turnover and collagen production, causing the skin to appear thin, wrinkled and dry.

- Cigarettes and free radicals, UV radiation, oxygen deprivation and neglect are the primary enemies of healthy, wrinkle-free and attractive skin.

- The aging process can be slowed to a crawl by adhering to a simple, consistent program of skin maintenance; Cleansing, Moisturizing and Exfoliating.

# Chapter 2: Saving Your Skin

## The Myth of Fancy Soap

The single purpose of a bar or a bottle of soap is to remove dirt and excess oil from the skin, penetrate and clean out porphyrins (bacterial poop) from the pores. This prepares the skin to receive the specific treatments and products that fit your skin type. Soaps and cleansers are supposed to clean your skin. Basic cleansing means washing your face every morning and every night at bedtime. Do that, and you're probably good to go.

Basic soap is not meant to moisturize, protect, or treat your skin. Once upon a time, in a land far, far away, selecting a brand of face soap was as easy as selecting a physician: most towns had just one.

My family used Ivory Soap because that's the brand my mom thought was purest and safest. The advertisements said that Ivory soap was "ninety nine and forty four one hundredths percent pure." Who could argue with that?

So the truth is out. I was "An Ivory Baby"!

In fact, if you use the proper moisturizer for your skin-type and apply sunscreen religiously, Ivory is still great soap. But things got complicated along the way. Through the years, we were bombarded with advertisements which led us to make "useless soap transitions;" i.e.: changing our cleanser brands because of flashy ads rather than because it made scientific sense.

## Pure, Mild IVORY SOAP
## Doctors' First Choice
### For Complexion Care

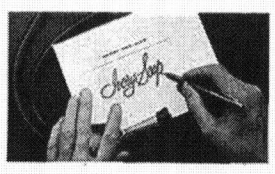

**Every practicing doctor in America** was recently mailed this question by a leading medical journal: "What soap is your first choice for skin care?" In the answers doctors, including skin doctors and baby doctors, voted: FIRST CHOICE... IVORY SOAP. Yes, Ivory first again! Why don't *you* try Ivory?

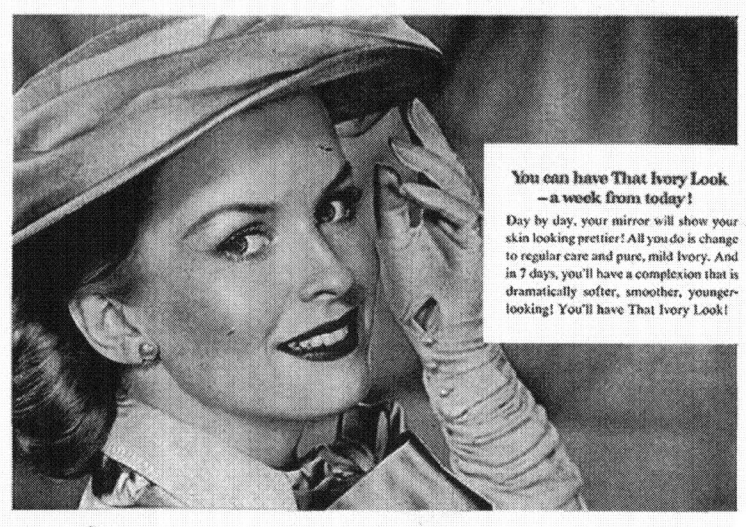

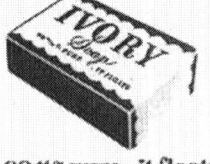

**You can have That Ivory Look — a week from today!**

Day by day, your mirror will show your skin looking prettier! All you do is change to regular care and pure, mild Ivory. And in 7 days, you'll have a complexion that is dramatically softer, smoother, younger-looking! You'll have That Ivory Look!

99 44/100% pure... it floats

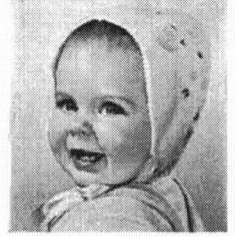

**Mild enough for a baby's skin!**

The milder the beauty soap, the better the condition of your skin — the prettier your complexion. And Ivory is mild enough for a baby's skin... doctors' first choice for her complexion and yours.

---

When Neutrogena first arrived in the grocery aisles, I switched because I liked its glycerin feel and amber transparency. Now, I've become a firm believer in Dove Extra Sensitive Skin. They are all good products.

Practically any gentle, non-deodorant, non-medicated soap is the perfect facial soap for more than 50% of us. Special soaps are for special problems -- excessively dry skin, oily skin, acne-prone skin -- but the rest of us can use just about any soap and look fine.

That's why I was so disturbed when a lovely, forty-something patient arrived at my office for a BOTOX® treatment. She had just come from an upscale boutique where a young salesgirl who had probably never had a blemish, line or wrinkle on her barely post-pubescent face convinced my patient that a $125 bar of Plank's Cor Soap was absolutely essential for her skincare routine.

That was not a typo; One Hundred and Twenty Five Dollars -- for soap.

I had been treating this patient for quite some time, and had always been impressed by her naturally beautiful complexion. She was told the Colloidal Silver in Plank's Cor Soap was anti-bacterial, and that the Sericin Silk extract would lock in moisture and keep out UV rays.

Why the antibacterial? In the three years I had been treating her, she'd never had a single pimple… not one. In addition, silk may block UV rays, but there is absolutely no UV protection offered by silk strands in soap, none whatsoever. After all, the pigment in silk drapes fades in the sun. Sericin Silk extract is meaningless nonsense.

Even if Cor soap possessed magical properties, for $125, it should sing and dance in the soap dish. Silver sells for about $18 an ounce. A bar of Cor weighs 4.4 ounces. For $125, you can buy a full seven ounces of 99.99% pure silver.

There are lots of excellent soaps on the market that will clean your face quite nicely. I use and recommend Dove Extra Sensitive Skin, which costs about $2.50 a bar.

## The Acid Mantle

The Acid Mantle is a thin, oily layer secreted by the sweat and sebaceous glands in the skin, and has a pH of approximately 5.

PH may be a bit of a mystery to many. Your high school science teacher probably explained it, but that seems like an eternity ago. Besides, who actually listened to teachers in high school when we were totally distracted discovering the opposite sex?

Here's the gist of pH: It's a way to measure acidity or alkalinity on a scale of 1 to 14, with a mid-point of 7. Water is a neutral substance, neither acidic nor alkaline, and therefore, has a pH of 7. Sulphuric acid has a very low pH; approximately pH-1. Caustic drain cleaner has the highest alkaline value with a pH of around 14.

On the pH scale of 1-14, the Acid Mantle of the skin is *mildly* acidic with a value of 5, but that level of acidity is enough to protect us from many infectious agents like *p. acnes* bacteria. The acid kills acne bacteria and neutralizes slightly alkaline chemical pollutants in the air to protect our skin from irritation and inflammation.

Soap has a pH of about 11 or 12. It is alkaline and, although its alkalinity helps wash the grime, makeup and body oil down the drain, it also temporarily reduces or removes the protection afforded by the Acid Mantle.

*Temporarily* is the operative word. We constantly replenish the acidity and restore the natural value of pH 5 to our skin. For a majority of people with non-acne prone, irritation-free, healthy skin, the use of regular old soap poses no problem and acidity in the skin is easily restored.

The rest of us need to buy cleansers that are slightly acidic, specifically formulated to preserve the Acid Mantle, but still provide adequate cleansing of the skin and pores.

Neutragena, Dermalogica or Mallon & Goetz products all fulfill this purpose. Mallon & Goetz, in particular, provides a complete line of affordable formulations for a wide variety of skin types, and are hard to equal from a qualitative standpoint.

## How Bad is Your Acne?

That's a very important question to ask before planning a course of acne treatment. Note the phrase "course of treatment," because acne is a persistent problem seldom totally cured. Pimples may come and go, but if you're one of those unfortunate people who are "acne prone," you're probably in for a prolonged, albeit intermittent, battle with the *p. acnes* bacteria.

Severe cystic acne, pustules and ongoing scarring, must be treated aggressively. Acne scars often become emotional scars. They can lead to social avoidance, and frustrating attempts to cover the damage with unsightly, thick cover-ups that only exacerbate the problem and lead to cycles of more acne, more scarring and more social avoidance. Never treat severe acne on your own. Consult a dermatologist, who is an acne specialist.

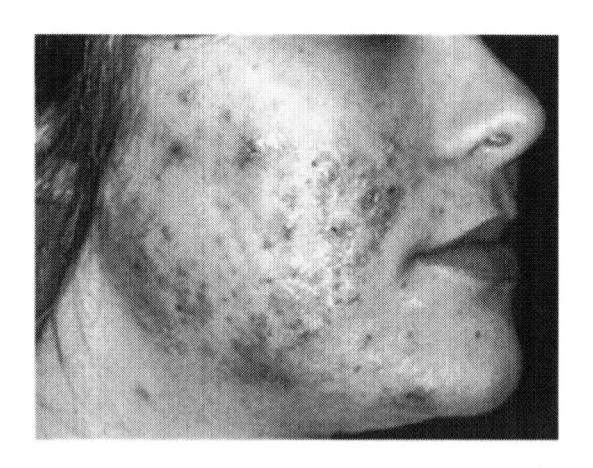

If the problem is moderate, with occasional breakout of "whiteheads" and "blackheads" but no acne scarring, more conservative treatment is indicated. A treatment program begins with weekly facials by a professional aesthetician to exfoliate, unclog and deeply clean the pores to remove debris.

A topical combination gel containing Clindamycin and Benzoyl Peroxide for use at bedtime is ideal. Clindamycin is a well established antibiotic that effectively kills *p. acnes*.

This bacterium breeds best in closed areas, such as clogged pores, and avoids oxygen rich environments. Benzoyl Peroxide introduces abundant oxygen into the pores, thereby killing the bacterium.

If your skin is too oily, cleansers or lotions containing Benzoyl Peroxide and/or Salicylic Acid make a good addition to the treatment plan. Salicylic Acid penetrates the follicles and pores and exfoliates (*i.e.*, removes) dead cells, thereby allowing oxygen and topical antibiotics to enter the pores and attack *p. acnes*. However, be careful the treatment isn't worse than the disease. Too much Bezoyl Peroxide and/or Salicylic Acid can dry your skin, making it more susceptible to infection and irritation. It's all about balance, which is another good reason you should consult an acne specialist.

If the problem is more persistent, a course of LED Blue Light or Photodynamic Therapy (PDT) with 5-aminolevulinic acid may be in order. (That's a mouthful. Just call it ALA). Light has many surprising effects. UV radiation can change DNA and cause cancer, but Red Light can sooth the skin and reduce inflammation, and Blue Light treatments soak the skin in specific light waves that inhibit the growth of *p. acnes*. Blue Light treatments take about twenty minutes, two or three times a week. Two months of treatment, accompanied by deep cleansing facials, provides a very effective alternative to antibiotic therapy for acne.

## Facials and Exfoliation

Skin takes a tremendous beating every day. Between the unavoidable assault of exhaust fumes, wind-swept dirt and grime, and particles and germs we inadvertently picked up on our hands before touching our face, our skin gets exposed to many things we'd rather not think about.

Adding to the problem is the fact that the natural oils in our skin are sticky and trap grit where ever it lands, and our pores are deep enough to shield some of this grit from even the most careful daily washing regimen.

Enter the aesthetician. There are some things you should leave in the hands of professionals, and exfoliation is one of them. There are about fifteen layers of dead cells on the skin surface. In order to replenish and stimulate new skin growth and open clogged pores, it's essential to remove these dead cells at frequent intervals.

The removal of dead skin cells is called exfoliation, and aestheticians are licensed and specially trained to perform this service. Whether they use a vibrating paddle (Vibraderm™) or the more common exfoliating devices which basically remove the dead cells by "sand blasting" them with a pressurized stream of tiny crystals (microdermabrasion), or perform a deep exfoliating facial with special scrubs or acids, the process should be performed at least every three months. I use the Vibraderm™ microdermabrasion unit because it's cleaner than blowing around tiny, messy crystals and every patient has his or her personal set of reusable paddles. I prefer clean and effective over messy and effective.

I strongly recommend a monthly facial during the two months between exfoliations. Facials provide exceptional cleansing and the opportunity for your aesthetician to evaluate the state of your skin and its production of oils, the effectiveness of your washing technique, and help you decide what products you should and should not be using. Bring along a list of all your skin care products and don't be shy. Choose an aesthetician as you would choose a physician -- carefully. Make sure he/she was trained at a recognized skincare academy, and works in a clean and hygienic spa or medical office.

Every physician has a favorite aesthetic school. Mine is Atelier Esthétique in New York City. I've never worked with better trained aestheticians.

## Moisturizers

The approximately fifteen layers of keratinized cells on the skin's surface keep the vast majority of moisturizers from ever reaching the deeper skin layers; a fact that sellers of cosmeceuticals simply ignore. Claims surrounding miracle ingredients, more effective penetration using "special molecular structure" and "proven anti-aging effects" are just unscientific hype.

That being said, you should moisturize twice a day, every day. "Wait!" you're thinking. "Didn't he just say moisturizers don't work?"

No. I said they don't effectively put moisture *into* your skin. Instead, a well chosen, inexpensive moisturizer acts like a protective coating and keeps the moisture you already have inside where it belongs. It will protect you from (among other things) losing moisture to dry air, excessive washing and abrasion by your pillow at night.

If you want moisture inside your skin, drink lots of water all year long. Dry winter winds rip moisture from your skin, and perspiration in warm weather or at the gym drains away precious water.

We seldom consider that dehydrating is caused by our normal bodily functions. However, we excrete approximately six cups of urine a day and lose four cups of water simply sweating and breathing. To prove this, try breathing into a clear plastic bag for a few breaths and you'll see the water condense on the inside. That's ten cups of water a day. Do you drink ten cups of replacement fluid a day? You should.

The question then becomes, "What constitutes a good moisturizer?" Look for products which are essentially natural, contain no unnecessary chemicals preservatives and no fragrances. Natural moisturizers may contain avocado, coconut oils, jojobas and other essential oils. If they contain aloe, make sure there are no aloe fibers dispersed in the product. A significant number of people develop allergic reactions to aloe fibers.

Check the label carefully. The natural moisturizing oil used will be listed among the first ingredients, along with certain alpha hydroxyl acids and beta hydroxyl acids incorporated to properly balance acidity. This added acidity is important to maintain the acid mantle which protects the skin from bacteria and free radicals in pollution.

Always remember the First Law of Skincare: More Expensive Does Not Always Mean Better.

## Sun Protection Factor

Selecting the right sunscreen is a bit more complex. SPF stands for "sun protection factor." Almost everyone has heard that SPF-30 is the upper limit of effectiveness. This is absolutely false. Sunscreens rated up to SPF-50 and higher are effective. Even the conservative FDA agrees with this claim. If you're planning a beach outing or a day in the summer sun, SPF-50 is the only way to go.

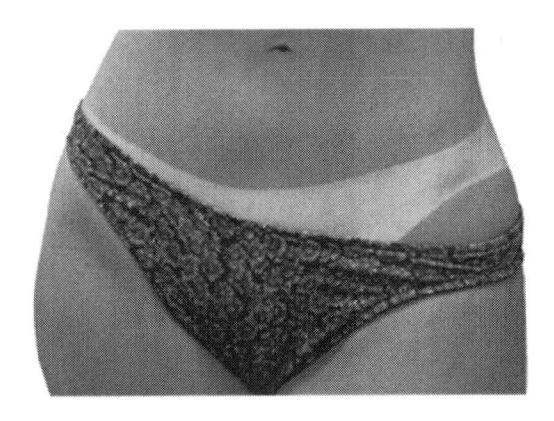

For year round use -- yes, year round -- SPF-15-30 is sufficient unless you have a very pale complexion. Both types of UV radiation, UVA and UVB, are hazardous to skin health. UVB causes surface sunburns and UVA affects deeper connective-tissue.

Both are just as dangerous in the winter as the summer. However, UV exposure is generally less intense in the winter because we are covered in clothes to keep us warm. If you're into winter sports like skiing or sledding, use SPF-50 on all exposed areas, and remember that UV radiation penetrates clouds and even window glass. Better safe than sorry.

Here's another thing I hear patients say all the time: "I don't need sunscreen. I'm only in the sun for ten minutes a day." I'm sorry to bring bad news, but UV damage is cumulative. Ten minutes a day is over an hour a week, which is fifty hours per year, which is like lying on the beach from sunrise to sunset for a full week. Use sunscreen every day, all year.

Don't forget to read the label before you buy any skincare product. Avoid sunscreens containing Oxybenzone, a potentially harmful, hormone-disrupting compound that can penetrate the skin and enter the bloodstream. Another dangerous ingredient is Retinyl Palmitate, a derivative of vitamin A found in about 40% of sunscreens. The FDA is investigating whether Retinyl Palmitate accelerates skin damage and increases skin cancer risk when applied to skin exposed to sunlight.

The best ingredients are those which stay on the surface of the skin. Avoid penetrating chemicals which, while they may block UV rays, may also damage your skin. Titanium dioxide and zinc oxide are natural mineral sunscreens that sit on top of the skin and effectively block both UVA and UVB rays.

## Recap

- The First Law of Skincare: More Expensive Does Not Always Mean Better.

- Simple soaps and cleansers such as Ivory, Dove and Neutrogena are safe and effective for 50% of us. The rest need carefully ph balanced soaps to protect the acid mantle.

- Moisturizers don't provide moisture. They prevent moisture from escaping. Drink plenty of water, and you'll have moist skin.

- Sun Protection Factor ratings up to 50 have been proven effective. Use some level of protection all year, and select natural sunscreens which do not penetrate the skin and block both UVA and UVB rays.

## Chapter 3: "If you keep making that face..."

### BOTOX® at 30?

Used responsibly, I cannot think of a single flaw in this wonderful product. If I were to start a religion honoring physical beauty, BOTOX® would be its sacrament. BOTOX® every four months from age thirty would be as significant an observance as Easter, Passover or Ramadan.

As noted previously, *active wrinkles* form when we move our faces, and *passive wrinkles* are visible all the time. The old wives' tale our mothers warned us about is true: "If you keep making that face, it will stay like that!" We move the facial muscles hundreds of times a day for many years, and this turns active wrinkles into passive wrinkles. The skin loses its elasticity and the lines don't go away anymore.

BOTOX® is specifically designed to treat active wrinkles, and *only* active wrinkles. The process is very simple. When we make a facial expression, the nerve that triggers the muscle to contract releases a chemical signal to start the contraction. BOTOX® interferes with the signal chemical, and by weakening the reaction of the underlying muscles, BOTOX® minimizes creasing of the overlying skin. That protects the Dermis from damage to existing collagen matrix and allows normal collagen production to maintain smooth, un-furrowed skin. Thus, BOTOX® staves off the *creation* of passive wrinkles by preventing the constant repetition of active wrinkling.

I recently overheard a conversation between two women, one in her mid-fifties, the other age thirty-four, in the salon where I get my hair cut.

The older woman asked about pink spots on the younger woman's forehead. She replied, "I just had my BOTOX® done this afternoon." The older woman was amazed. "BOTOX? You're way too young for BOTOX," she said. I couldn't help but smile when the younger woman replied matter-of-factly, "I'm thirty-four. When I'm fifty, I won't have a wrinkle on my face." I thought to myself, "Smart girl."

BOTOX® is an amazing product, and despite rumors to the contrary, extremely safe. In fact, when a physician injects sixty units of BOTOX® into your facial muscles, you are exposed to something less dangerous than taking two extra strength aspirin for a headache. It is that safe. It is also an invaluable tool in the battle against visible signs of aging.

That said, it must be injected only by a trained professional. I've seen the results of poorly placed BOTOX® and they are not pretty. Try to avoid "discount BOTOX® deals." In the final analysis, you're not really paying for the BOTOX®; you're paying for the experience and expertise of the hand holding the syringe.

The goal is even distribution and unaltered facial symmetry, affecting only the specific muscles you've chosen to treat. Like any other treatment, BOTOX® requires careful clinical evaluation of each individual patient's needs. After all, no two patients have the same pattern of facial muscles anymore than they have the same biceps or abdominal muscles.

In planning BOTOX® treatments, a trained professional should ask the patient to raises his/her brow to see active brow lines; frown to evaluate the "11s"; and smile or squint to evaluate the Crow's Feet. I always take a few photos before starting a treatment.

Many physicians will mark out his/her injection plan on your face by drawing small dots with white eyeliner to pinpoint exactly where each injection will be most effective. A tiny needle called a "31 gauge" should be used to minimize bruising. I like to keep a "BOTOX® Map" of each patient's face. That way I can evaluate the effectiveness of the amount I used, measured in 'units,' in each area.

If your doctor just fills a syringe and starts injecting, run.

## BOTOX® Tx FLOW SHEET

NAME: *Jane Doe*

| 2cc/100U AREA | 1U/0.02cc UNITS |
|---|---|
| FRONTALIS | 13  17 |
| GLABELLA | 17 |
| CROW'S FEET | 9 / 9 |
| LIPS | |
| DAOs | / |
| PLATYSMA | / |
| OTHER | |

TREATMENT DATE: 01 / 20 / 12

INITIAL TX: BLACK
TOUCHUP : RED

The following photos show the most common BOTOX® treatment sites.

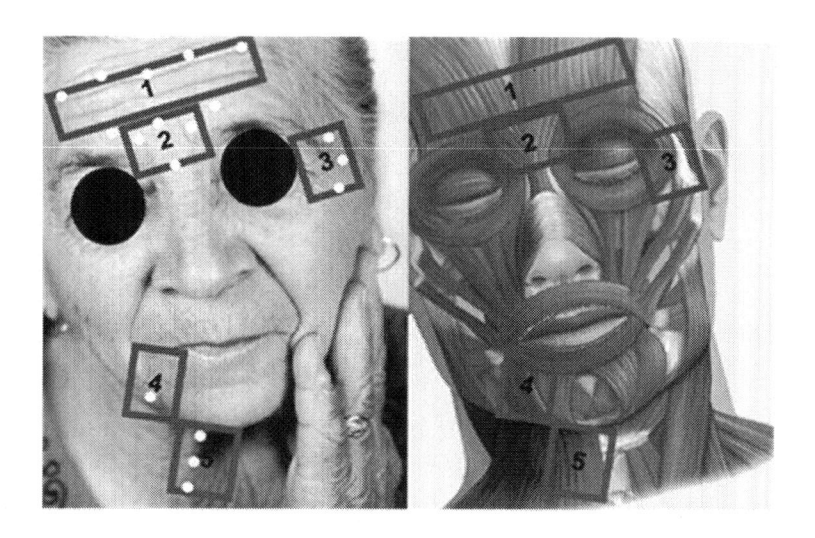

The photo on the left show the injection sites marked as white dots, and the picture on the right shows the corresponding muscles affected. Area 1, Brow Lines; Area 2, Glabella Lines, also known as "The Elevens"; Area 3, Crow's Feet; Area 4, DAO (Depressor of the Angle of the Mouth) and Area 5, Platysma Neck Bands.

Two areas deserve special mention. Area 4, the DAO, is a triangular muscle which pulls down the corner of the mouth. As we age, all the facial muscles naturally weaken, including the muscles that lift the corners of the mouth. Gravity also provides a downward pull. Weakening the DAO with a small amount of BOTOX allows the mouth to turn slightly upward again and lessens the appearance of constant sadness or scowling.

Area 5, the Platysma Band, is actually a border where the two sides of the Platysma Muscle once joined at the midline of the neck. As we age, the midline connection weakens and that telltale vertical band appears. By injecting BOTOX® into this band, we allow it to relax back towards the neck and become much less noticeable.

BOTOX® isn't cheap, and you can make it last longer and be more effective if you avoid lying down for a few hours after injection. That way the injection stays where it was placed until it settles in. Make as many facial expressions as possible in the first hour following an application of BOTOX®. The muscles will receive a smoother, more even distribution of BOTOX® rather than a large concentration at the injection site. You may look a bit strange walking down the street squinting and frowning at nothing (although in New York, no one will notice and you'll blend right in with other weirdoes talking and gesturing to themselves).

## Fillers Fill. That's All They Do

Fillers are designed to fill in defects and furrows *after* active wrinkles have become passive wrinkles. At that point, BOTOX® alone will no longer make the wrinkles disappear. BOTOX® will certainly stop your furrows from getting worse but, short of cosmetic surgery, fillers are the only way to lessen the appearance of existing damage and deep furrows.

Juvederm®, Restylane™ and Radiesse™, are the best known fillers. Juvederm® and Restylane™ consist of essentially the same compound, Hyaluronic Acid (HA), the most important natural space-filling substance in the human body. HA traps water to keep collagen hydrated, supple, and "youthful." An interesting fact: the composition of HA is identical in every mammalian species. That means that HA from my Miniature Schnauzer could be injected into my skin, causing no allergic reaction.

The difference between Juvederm® and Restylane™, and the several varieties of each, is the shape and size of the HA molecule clusters. The smaller the cluster, the more fluid it is and the more easily the physician can smooth the appearance of the injected filler. Different variations of Juvederm® and Restylane™ are reportedly better for different applications, but practitioners generally try different products and stick with the ones they like. I stopped using Restylane™ because the syringes were difficult and occasionally broke during application. I especially like Juvederm® Ultra 4 because it has a small amount of Lidocaine which helps diminish discomfort during injection.

Application of topical and/or injectible anesthesia is also a good idea when treating a patient with fillers. The placement of HA must be precise, balanced and even. If the patient is squirming around in pain during the treatment, the physician cannot possibly mirror the patient's every twist and turn. The result of uncontrolled movement during injection will be areas of unsightly bumps, irregularities and bruises.

Unfortunately, many practitioners have a cavalier attitude towards your pain, and the application of topical anesthesia takes up valuable office time. Hence, remember the Second

Law of Skincare: There's No Excuse for Inadequate Pain Control -- Ever.

**Juvederm®**
The following photo is marked with the most common uses of Juvederm®. The numbered furrows are easily filled and results are generally excellent with this product.

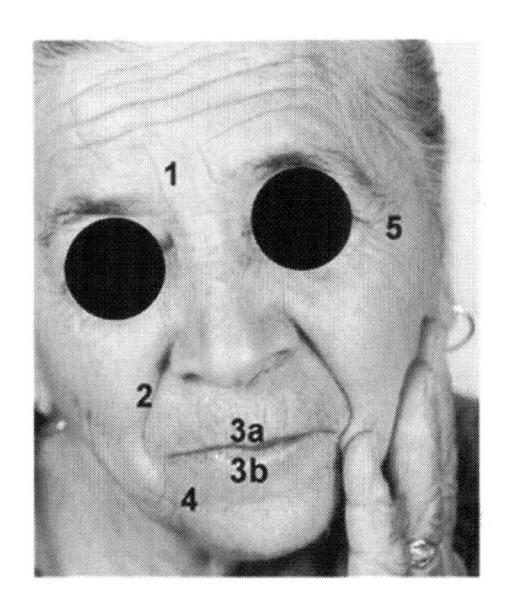

Number 1 marks "The Elevens," an excellent place to begin discussion of fillers. Even if you wear your hair in bangs, these lines are always visible. A small amount of Juvederm® injected properly can virtually erase the Elevens. It's a fast and easy fix.

Number 2, the Nasolabial Folds (NLF), become deep for two reasons. First, they are the "Laugh Lines". Every time we smile or laugh they are accentuated and (fortunately) no sane physician would dream of using BOTOX® to stop you from smiling. The second reason the NLF deepen is subcutaneous volume loss. Our skin does not get looser and baggier as we age; rather, the tissue under our skin which keeps it stretched and in place begins to disappear. We lose fat and muscle from our faces as we age, so the skin appears to sag.

To see how this works, inflate a balloon and put it in a safe place for a week. Slowly, the air will seep out no matter how tightly it's tied. The rubber surface, smooth and tight while the balloon was fully inflated, will now appear wrinkled and flaccid, just like your face once the fat and muscle begin to disappear.

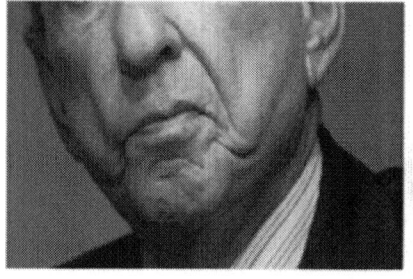

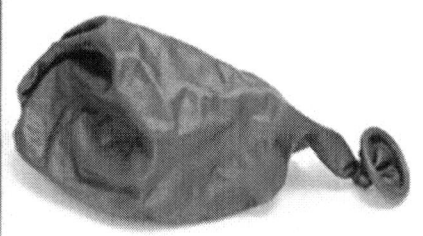

Area 3a is just above the upper lip. People who spent a lot of time in the sun, smoked for years or lost their upper teeth are especially prone to multiple vertical lip lines. Just look in a mirror while you suck on a straw to see these lines form. Smoke twenty cigarettes a day for 10-20 years and imagine the result. Remember, "If you keep making that face…"

Area 3b represents the actual lips. The upper lip is especially prone to age-related volume loss and, along with it, the loss of that voluptuous pouty look. After carefully numbing the lip area, dramatic changes can be made with a single syringe of Juvederm®. Fuller lips look younger and sexier.

Remember that the goal is sexy, not clownish. You can always have the doctor add more filler later, but removing excessive filler after treatment is nearly impossible. You'll be stuck with lips that don't fit your face for 5-6 months. Remember the Third Law of Skincare: The Worst Enemy of "Good" is "Better". (That's a pretty good motto for life, in general, too.)

If you're undergoing a procedure and the practitioner says, "That looks pretty good", then it's time to stop injecting. "Pretty good" is a good place to stop. You can always come back for more. Here's what happens when too much is used at one time.

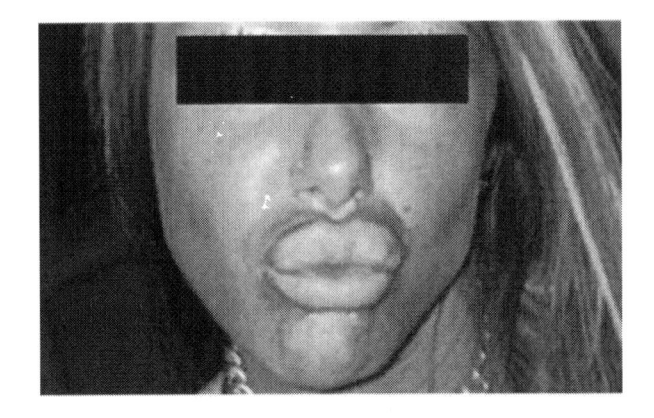

I use Juvederm® for areas 4 and 5, the Marionette Lines and Crow's Feet.

## Radiesse® and the "Liquid Face Lift"

Radiesse® is not only more widely useful than other fillers; it also lasts 18-24 months.

The beauty of Radiesse® is its versatility and double impact. Young skin contains collagen which gives it volume, flexibility and strength. As we age, collagen breaks down, our muscles and fat diminish, and facial volume is lost. Radiesse wrinkle filler not only fills defects, its unique formulation stimulates "collagenesis" – the production of new collagen – which results in restored facial volume and natural looking wrinkle correction that lasts.

Radiesse® is used to perform a "Liquid Face Lift." By carefully placing precise quantities of this product along the cheekbones, jaw line, nasolabial folds and marionette lines, your physician can replace significant amounts of tissue volume which has been lost with age. The process fills out the skin and facial contours, both smoothing and tightening.

On the left side of the following illustration, the black arrows labeled as "vectors" mark the direction we want to pull, tighten and lift the skin. The object of the injections is to elevate the cheekbone area and pull back the nasolabial folds and fill the jaw line to tighten and repair the jowls.

On the right, the gray arrows and gray X-marks indicate where Radiesse® typically is placed, although the exact amount is based entirely on the needs of the specific patient. This is an art, not a science, and definitely not a cookie cutter process for the inexperienced practitioner.

The three lines marked in white are at the "pre-jowl sulcus." It is the indentation where the front of the jowl meets the back of the chin. This area requires special attention because properly filling it leaves a smooth line in place of the unsightly depression that ruins the lower facial contour.

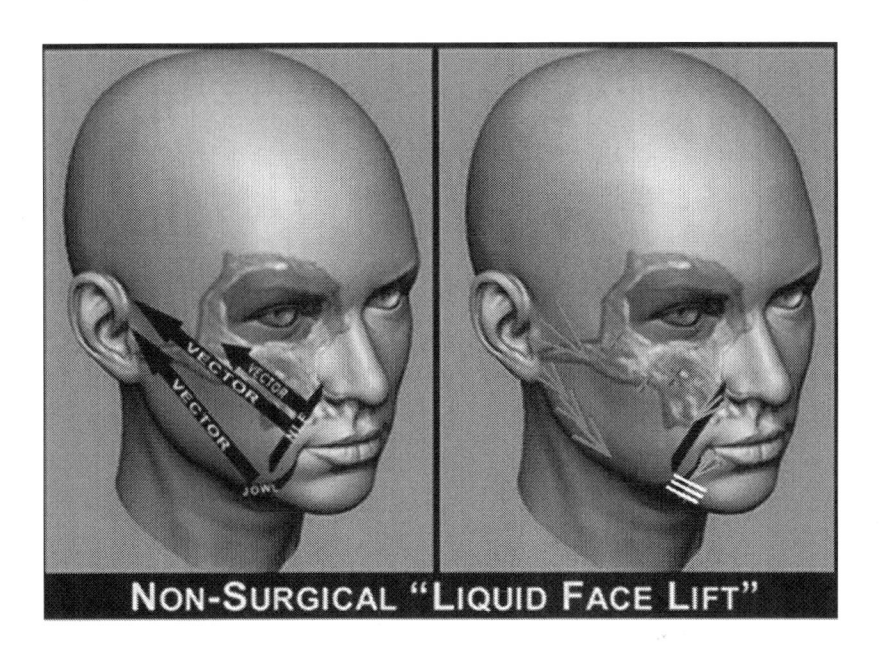

**NON-SURGICAL "LIQUID FACE LIFT"**

The upper portion of the nasolabial fold – the triangular indentation next to the nostril – is generally deeper and requires extra Radiesse®, as does the upper, triangular portion of the marionette line.

The results of properly placed fillers are immediate, virtually pain free, and provide a natural appearing lift that is smooth and full. This is a stark contrast to the often over-tightened, plastic-appearing result of a surgical facelift.

A Liquid Facelift takes about three hours. Afterward, the patient should stay home and ice the area for a day. One day of social downtime to ice your face is a small price to pay for the wonderful effect of this exciting new procedure.

## Recap

- The Second Law of Skincare: There's No Excuse for Inadequate Pain Control -- Ever.

- The Third Law of Skincare: The Worst Enemy of "Good" is "Better".

- BOTOX® relaxes muscle contractions by blocking the nerve's chemical signal. It is amazingly safe, and effectively treats active wrinkles so you never get passive wrinkles.

- Juvederm® is a hypoallergenic filler for passive wrinkles. It smoothes and fills areas such as the nasolabial folds and is the filler of choice for lip enhancement.

- Radiesse® lasts 18-24 months, fills large areas, and has the additional benefit of forming new collagen. It is the key ingredient in a Liquid Facelift which results in a tightened, smoother, more attractive and youthful facial contour.

# Chapter 4: The Light Fantastic

## Photo-Thermo-Lysis

Every patient knows a place where he/she can get unwanted hair removed. It's sort of a rite of passage to never again have to shave your under arms, legs and bikini area. Every spa and laser center has aestheticians performing this valuable service, and the results are usually acceptable.

There is, however, one simple exception which deserves comment: the Big Lie. Anyone who tells you that white hair or light blond hair can be removed with a laser, or any other light based device, is lying. Period.

I teach laser technique at spas and physician's offices. At one particularly busy spa, the owner and managers demanded the aestheticians sell packages of laser hair removal to blond and white-haired people. These unscrupulous businessmen duped and bullied the aestheticians into believing this result could be achieved with their "new improved laser." A revolt ensued after my seminar. Aestheticians generally are sincerely interested in their clients' well being, and these women simply refused to sell any more of these packages to blond or white-haired clients.

Needless to say, I wasn't invited back to teach there again.

Lasers and light-based treatments (flash lamps) do not work on light colored or white targets. The reason is logical and scientific. In the case of hair removal, light (Photo) is absorbed by the melanin pigment in hair and converted into heat (Thermo), which destroys (Lysis) the hair follicle. The darker the target hair, the hotter it will get when light hits it; hence the term Photo-thermo-lysis.

Essentially, there are two types of light-based devices; True Lasers and Flash Lamps. Lasers produce only one, exact frequency of light. They are very selective and target only one color target. Flash Lamps are just that – lamps, and are akin to the light bulbs in your home because they produce many frequencies of light. Different flash lamps produce different frequency ranges, but the idea is the same, and the target range is always broader for a lamp than it is for a laser.

The white arrow in the figure below represents a single frequency laser - in this case a 532 YAG Laser - which generates only one frequency and color of light. The flash lamp, on the other hand, generates a wide range of frequencies from 620-770 and affects several different color targets.

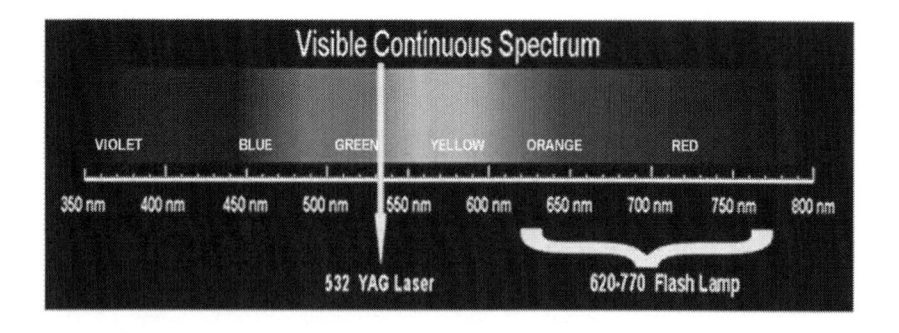

**Visible Continuous Spectrum**

| VIOLET | BLUE | GREEN | YELLOW | ORANGE | RED |
|--------|------|-------|--------|--------|-----|
| 350 nm  400 nm | 450 nm  500 nm | 550 nm  600 nm | 650 nm  700 nm | 750 nm  800 nm |

532 YAG Laser            620-770 Flash Lamp

Every color is a different frequency of light and, therefore, each lamp or laser target is different and specific.

Every Woman's Guide to Anti-Aging Medicine

The practitioner is responsible for selecting the correct laser or light-based device for your specific problem area. A practitioner cannot use the same laser to get rid of brown spots or hair as they would use to remove red or purple spider veins.

Photothermolysis is an easy concept to prove. We wear white in summer to reflect rather than absorb sunlight to stay cool. Do a simple experiment: place a sheet of white paper and a sheet of black paper in the sun. The black paper will absorb a lot of light and heat up rapidly. The white paper will reflect light and may not heat up at all.

It's exactly the same for laser hair removal. Light brown hair is difficult to remove, and blond or white hair is almost impossible to remove.

If you have those fine, tiny hairs in your face, it's even worse. Imagine putting a thin black thread in the sun and a sheet of black paper. The paper has much more surface area and therefore absorbs more light. The thread has limited surface area may not heat up at all. That's why fine hairs are much more difficult to destroy with lasers and flash lamps than thick, coarse hair.

Today, the Brazilian total pubic hair removal is all the rage. Many women believe their mates find pubic hairlessness to be sexy and attractive. However, in the course of your adult life styles may change and therefore a certain amount of pubic hair may become the new "in look." Better to go with a modified Brazilian which leaves a "Landing Strip" of hair about one inch wide. It will always be easy to shave a one inch strip and, no matter how skimpy the bikini, the hair will never be seen. Meanwhile, you leave open your aesthetic options in the future.

## Tightening and Resurfacing the Skin with Light

There are five main systems of skin tightening devices. The first system uses Radio Frequency (RF). Thermage™ is the biggest player in the RF arena. In my opinion, Thermage™ is very painful - more painful than any other systems discussed here - and the results it produces are just not as good. In one questionnaire of Thermage™ patients, 60% were dissatisfied with the result. That pretty well sums it up. No Thermage for my patients.

Radio Frequency has a definite place in the facial cosmetic tool kit, but not for skin tightening. RF surgical systems like the Ellman Surgitron® Dual RF™ provide virtually bloodless incisions and a faster recovery time for many facial procedures. They are especially good for eyelid surgery.

The second system is the very popular Fraxel® treatment. Fraxel® was the first "fractional" laser system on the market and, as such, rapidly became synonymous with skin tightening and resurfacing. Fractional means that the laser beam is divided into many, separate and smaller beams of light. The Fraxel® name is to fractional lasers what Xerox™ is to copiers. It may or may not be the best, but it's certainly the most recognized.

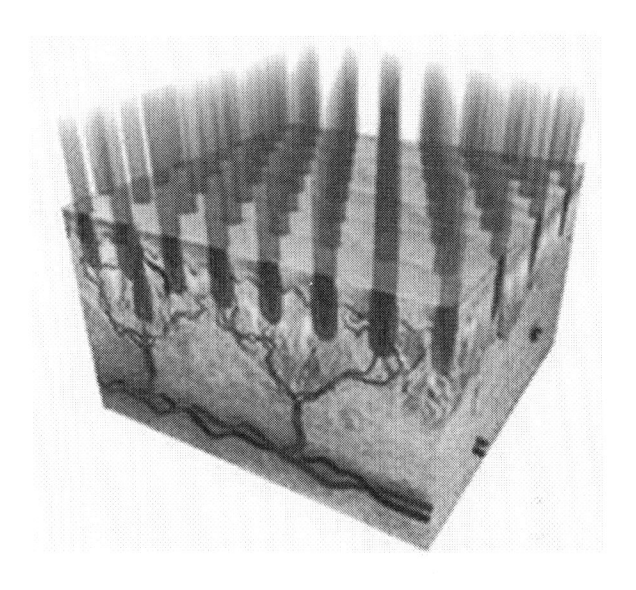

As the laser beam heats its target, it creates "islands of damage" with the expectation that, as these tiny areas heal, the skin will develop new collagen and become tighter.

At the same time, Fraxel™ promises rejuvenation, reversal of sun damage, and improvement of skin texture and aging lines. That's a tall and often unfulfilled expectation. One Fraxel™ treatment is usually not sufficient, and each treatment costs between $2,500-5,000. Sometimes, physicians recommend 4-5 treatments which can become very expensive. Name recognition, not effectiveness, is responsible for the exorbitant price of Fraxel™.

Fraxel™ treatments are also very hot and invasive. More patients arrive at my office burned by a Fraxel™ than any other device, and the potential for complications increases when hurried physicians do several different procedures at once.

I evaluated a lovely woman whose physician simultaneously transplanted fat into her temple area and immediately Fraxeled the skin over the fat grafts. The laser melted the fat and the combination of surface and sub-dermal heat burned *both* sides of the skin. The result was a serious infection and several areas of hair loss.

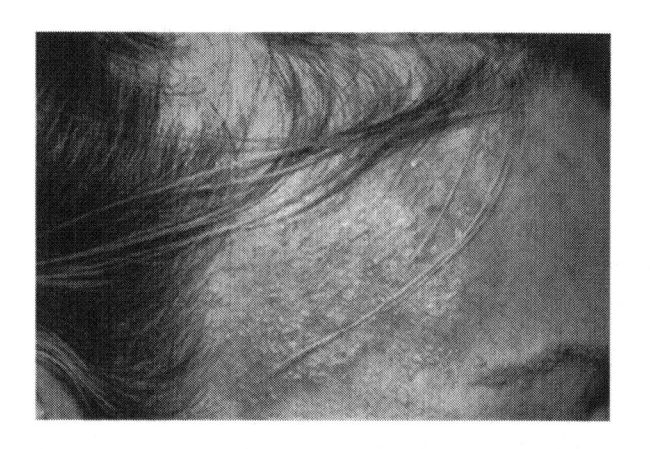

To make matters worse, every few years a "new generation Fraxel™" is brought onto the market and patients, swayed by media rather than clinical results, want the newest version of the laser they saw on a TV morning show or read about in a woman's magazine. This spurs practitioners to rush out and buy the newest machine before sufficient evidence exists to justify the "improved" treatment.

In 2006, I was offered a "special deal" at the Anti-Aging Medical Conference: I could purchase a new Fraxel™ for just $99,000. Five years later, used Fraxel™ machines in perfect condition sell for about $25,000. Obviously not a good investment, and not good for patients to whom the price of new equipment is passed on as elevated medical fees.

The third system, Ultrasound Tightening, arrived on the market with much accompanying fanfare. Unfortunately, the studies are weak, at best. Treatment is delivered via a focused ultrasound device that lays down rows of small thermal coagulation zones (similar to fractional, but not laser).

In one study, patients were given ultrasound brow lifts and the results were then analyzed by three experienced clinicians unaware of the method of treatment. At ninety days after treatment, 86% of patients were judged to have clinically "significant" eyebrow elevation. Average eyebrow lift was 1.7 mm. All subjects developed trace to slight edema (swelling) and erythema (redness) that lasted a week.

What that means in practical terms is that all the patients were red for a week, and got an average improvement of 6/100ths of an inch. Laymen might think it odd that clinicians dared to describe this miniscule change as "significant."

The fourth system is a combination treatment, and the one I use most frequently in my office. It's time tested, safe, requires 4-5 days of social downtime, and actually works. I always treat the deep tissue (the Dermis), first and the superficial layer (the Epidermis) second. Improving the quality of skin is similar in concept to building a house. Finish the foundation before starting the roof.

The first stage of this system involves 2-3 treatments with a TITAN™ laser, separated by three weeks and then followed by a single procedure every 6-8 months. I am a hands-on laser practitioner and perform all advanced laser procedures myself; I never rely on a laser technician.

TITAN™ uses a safe, infrared light to heat the Dermis well below the skin's surface. The heat is focused on the Dermis, while the Epidermis is protected through continuous cooling with the TITAN™ hand piece.

I add two essential ingredients to the treatment regimen: cold gel spread over the skin to further protect the patient, and forty-five minutes of topical anesthetic. I repeat: A doctor's office should be a *pain free zone*.

The beauty of TITAN™ is that it only promises one thing – tightening – and it delivers.

The intense, deep heat produced by the TITAN™ works in two ways. Fresh collagen strands are coiled and tight, while older collagen strands are looser and uncoiled. TITAN™ heating re-coils and tightens old collagen strands quite effectively. Collagen-producing fibroblast cells are stimulated to produce more collagen by any form of damage, whether real or "perceived" by the tissue. TITAN™ essentially fools the fibroblasts into believing they've been burned, even though the heat is safely below the burn threshold. The result is production of fresh, new collagen and subsequent, progressive skin tightening over a six-week period.

There is no down time after the initial TITAN™ treatments on the Dermis. I can perform a PEARL™ laser resurfacing treatment on the Epidermis as little as 2 weeks later.

The PEARL™ also reduces pigmentation spots, sun damage and fine surface wrinkles. If additional treatment is warranted, another PEARL™ can be performed as soon as four weeks later. In my experience, about 80% of my patients are satisfied with two treatments with a TITAN™ laser and a single PEARL™ treatment.

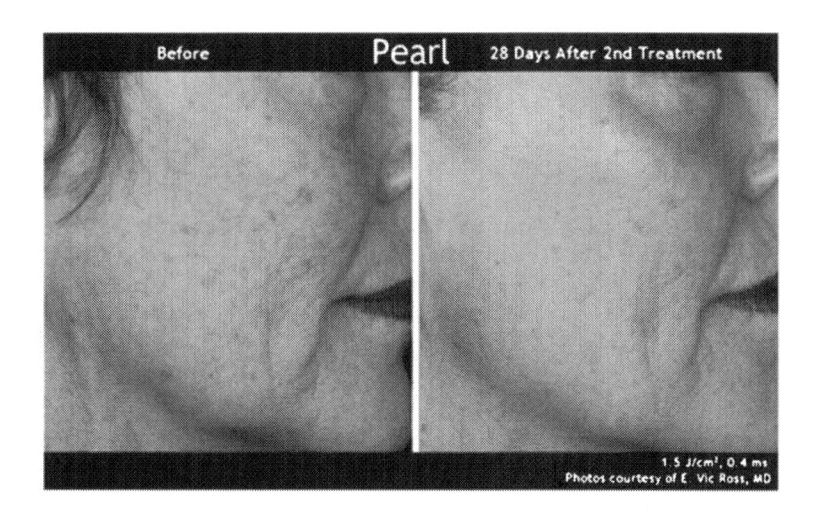

Before | Pearl | 28 Days After 2nd Treatment

1.5 J/cm², 0.4 ms
Photos courtesy of E. Vic Ross, MD

The PEARL™ laser vaporizes the upper epidermal layers without oozing or peeling. The vaporized cells are gone. For four days, patients are instructed to smear Aquaphor on their skin and new skin grows underneath the Aquaphor. It's a very elegant technique, though admittedly, Aquaphor can be a bit messy. After the PEARL™ laser treatment, patients are very pink and may experience a bit of swelling, but by day five they have usually fully recovered.

The fifth and newest system is a fractionated Carbon Dioxide ($CO_2$) Laser. Older, non-fractionated $CO_2$ lasers were once the gold standard for skin tightening and resurfacing. That was years before other modalities came to market. While the old $CO_2$ lasers worked amazingly well in the right hands, few practitioners were sufficiently skilled and therefore the risks were unacceptably high. Patients were frequently burned or scarred and, as more sophisticated lasers arrived, $CO_2$ lasers fell from grace.

Recently, however, $CO_2$ technology has changed with the introduction of the DEKA SmartXide DOT $CO_2$ laser. In a single system, it offers the versatility of both deep and superficial skin resurfacing and very reliable skin tightening, in one treatment with 4-5 days of recovery time.

Every parameter of the DEKA SmartXide is easily adjustable, and able to treat patients with problems as simple as enlarged pores or as complex as extreme acne scarring.

## Spot Treatment
Many patients don't need full resurfacing. They may only have pigmented spots from sun damage on the face, chest (décolleté) and arms. These spots are almost universally brown in color, and caused by repeated sun exposure and sun burn, or "post-inflammatory hyper-pigmentation." That may seem like a mouthful, but it's simple to explain. *Post-inflammatory* means something occurring after-inflammation, and *hyper-pigmentation* means the development of increased pigmented spots in a specific area.

Most practitioners consider IPL (Intense Pulsed Light) the best method for treating this type of problem. A light frequency is selected which specifically targets brown spots while leaving the normal, surrounding skin undamaged.

All laser and light-based skin treatments must be supervised or performed by a physician. This cannot be stressed too strongly. In too many spas, licensed aestheticians with little laser experience employ potentially dangerous machines without proper, medical supervision.

Some spas even employ "Laser Technicians" or laser techs. Virtually anyone can become a laser tech. You don't even need a high school diploma to qualify. Laser tech schools are multiplying like rabbits and, after a course as short as *four weeks*, laser techs are set loose on an unsuspecting public to wield lasers and lamps which have the potential to burn or even permanently scar your skin.

Some states like New Jersey limit the use of lasers to physicians. Remember the Fourth Law Of Skincare: A Physician Should Be Present While Your Laser Procedure Is Performed. A physician's expertise is essential to deal with any unexpected problems. "Present in the office" means readily available, not on the other side of town.

## Lasers and People of Color

It is important to dispel an erroneous belief from the distant past. (In laser terms, "distant past" means about ten years.) Let it be known throughout the land that People of Color *can* have safe, effective laser treatments.

In laser terms, People of Color not only refers to African Americans, but also darker-skinned Latinos, Middle Easterners, and most Asians. Because of all that extra melanin, however, they require special care and specially trained practitioners.

Laser technology has progressed light years (pardon the pun) over the last decade, and more physicians are taking the time to learn the principles that apply to treating darker skin. Physicians need to choose the correct real laser -- not flash lamp -- and then start treatments at substantially lower power settings than those used to treat Caucasian skin.

During each treatment, it is important to carefully observe the skin reaction to ascertain the burn threshold for each individual patient. This is another reason that People of Color should only be treated under the direct supervision of a physician. Treatment requires extensive training and clinical expertise, and generally aestheticians and laser techs are not up to the task.

Flash lamps such as IPL treatments and non-laser flash lamp hair removal are out of the question for People of Color. As noted previously, flash lamps produce many frequencies of light and therefore pose an unacceptable risk of burning darker skinned patients.

Hair reduction can easily be performed with a laser on People of Color. I use the Cutera CoolGlide™ 1064 because it is a very accurate and adjustable machine.

African American men and some post-menopausal African American women tend to grow very thick, curly facial hair. This hair is so curled that it often becomes ingrown and infected. The problem resembles infected follicles, and is called Pseudo Folliculitis Barbi (PFB), Latin for "false follicle infection of the beard." It is a common, well recognized problem in the African American community and has a nickname, "the nubs." Unfortunately, many dermatologists and general practitioners treat only the infection, as though it were a case of acne, without treating the underlying cause.

Patients with the nubs require full hair removal in the affected area to prevent the problem from recurring. In male patients, it is wise to leave the moustache and chin hair undisturbed, as men may want to grow a goatee or moustache at a later date. Fortunately, these two areas are neither as often nor as severely affected as the neck, jaw line and cheeks.

A secondary problem in People of Color is that when they suffer from acne or PFB they develop excessive pigmentation at the infection site. This is called Post-Inflammatory Hyper-pigmentation (PIH). The following before-and-after photo demonstrates how severe PIH can become.

I treated this patient six times with a CoolGlide™ laser to remove the hair follicles, and then every three weeks for a year to destroy the excess pigment. We were both thrilled with the result.

**LASER TREATMENT INGROWN HAIR & SCAR PIGMENT**

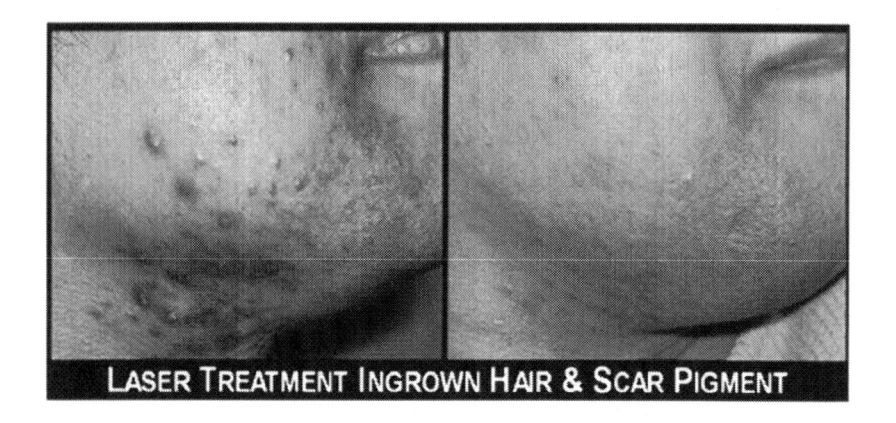

Skin tightening with a TITAN™ also works well on People of Color. The infrared light source can be adjusted for every patient. Very safe, effective tightening can be accomplished on virtually anyone of any skin tone with this device.

However, dark skinned patients should not be peeled, with either lasers or chemicals, as it can lead to severe PIH and awful patterns of pigment changes.

## Recap

- The Fourth Law of Skincare: A Physician Should Be Present While Your Procedure Is Performed.

- Laser and light-based treatments get the best results when the unit selected treats only one problem at a time. Your skin is not a place to multi-task.

- The best skin tightening system is, hands down, Cutera's TITAN™. It is tried and true.

- PEARL™ treatments resurface the skin with minimal downtime and also remove spots and fine wrinkles.

- IPL is the gold standard for post-inflammatory hyper-pigmentation to remove sun-damaged brown spots.

- Dark skinned patients can be safely and successfully treated with lasers, provided the proper laser and correct adjustments are made to accommodate dark skin's increased absorption of light.

## Chapter 5: Hormonal High Jinks

Hormone Replacement Therapy (HRT) is a very controversial topic within the medical community. Many reputable practitioners refuse to even consider HRT. Certain hormones have been linked to cancer in susceptible patients, and all hormones can cause side effects.

That being said, careful patient selection, thorough follow-up evaluation, and frequent laboratory reports are far better than total avoidance of such a useful treatment option. Too many women are denied access to HRT even though they would never experience cancers or other side effects.

Another, more insidious factor tarnishes the reputation of HRT. There are more than a few "medical offices" which are really just "Hormone Mills." They are staffed by physicians who prescribe hormones as if they were M&Ms. Little or no blood testing is performed, no routine follow-up appointments are made, and patients are left to pray their dosages are correct, which too often is the exception and not the rule. *Most of the bad press HRT receives is directly related to the sloppy practice of medicine* and, unfortunately, conscientious and careful physicians prescribing HRT are often wrongfully tarred with the same brush.

HRT is an area where medical science and medical practice are years apart, and as a result, women suffer the consequences in premature aging and diminished quality of life. There are numerous, influential studies clearly demonstrating the benefits of HRT, yet very few physicians who prescribe and manage it. It is hard to know whether they are afraid of the risk to their patients or simply too conservative to take the next step into the future of medicine.

The risk of complications from HRT is further decreased when bio-identical, topical hormone creams are prescribed in lieu of synthetic hormones. Bio-identical hormones are exactly like your natural hormones. They are absorbed into the blood stream and can be dosed much more controllably than oral medications. Artificial "estrogen-like" compounds or estrogens derived from horse urine should be avoided altogether. Women deserve better.

Treatment should begin with very low dosing, and doses increased only after blood work demonstrates the need. Mistakes are human and unavoidable. If practitioners start by doing less than necessary, it is always possible to adjust the dose upward.

Hence, the First Law Of Hormone Replacement Therapy: HRT Takes Time. It Is A Process, Not An Event.

When most of us think of hormones, Estrogen, Progesterone and Testosterone are the first that come to mind. These three receive the most media attention because they are known as the "sex hormones," and we all know how much the press likes to feature anything containing the word "sex."

## Estrogen
Each of these three sex hormones is produced by the ovaries and plays an important role in maintaining adult female health, happiness and vitality.

When menstrual cycles are regular and reliable, hormonal mood swings can be predicted in most cases. Girls reach puberty (from the Latin *pubertas*, which means adulthood) at different ages, although the average age for initial breast development is 10½ years and menstruation typically begins at 12½. At puberty, secondary sexual changes occur, fertility is achieved, and skeletal growth is completed.

Both males and females have all three sex hormones, although pubescent girls have substantially higher levels of Estrogen than pubescent boys. This fact explains, in part, why girls experience earlier growth spurts than boys and why they stop growing earlier than boys. Both ends of our long bones (for example; legs, arms and fingers) have areas called the *epiphyses*. It is at these points, the growth plates of the epiphysis, where bones elongate as we grow. Higher Estrogen levels cause the growth plates to close sooner.

Throughout a woman's life, Estrogen is an important stimulant for bone growth and maintenance, while lack of Estrogen can lead to bone loss and fractures.

**Arm Bones at Wrist**

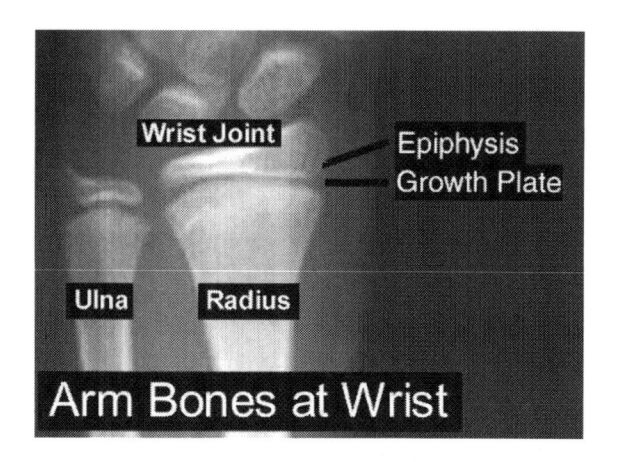

(X-ray showing Wrist Joint, Epiphysis Growth Plate, Ulna, Radius)

Most hormone levels decline relatively slowly over many years, which is what happens with Testosterone, Thyroid Hormone and Growth Hormone, all of which are discussed in later chapters. Menopause, on the other hand, is a precipitous drop in Estrogen and Progesterone and a fairly short term event. A woman can have completely normal hormonal levels in January, still experience regular periods, and become profoundly hormone deficient by December.

Menopausal symptoms vary from mildly uncomfortable to extremely difficult, and generally include some level of vaginal dryness, mood swings and hot flashes. Few women are fortunate enough to remain asymptomatic altogether.

Though the symptoms are seldom dangerous, they are often *very* upsetting and limiting. Hot flashes are often the worst symptom of menopause. About 60% of menopausal woman will suddenly experience the sensation of extreme heat accompanied by a red, flushed face and profuse sweating. Hot flashes can recur unexpectedly many times a day. Estrogen replacement is the treatment of choice.

Vaginal dryness during sexual stimulation is another frequent symptom, and experienced by 80% of menopausal women. Due to the pain and irritation of vaginal dryness, many women avoid sexual intercourse entirely. The men in their lives, unfamiliar with the symptoms of menopause, may erroneously believe their mates have lost interest in sex or are simply no longer excited by them.

Estrogen is responsible for vaginal lubrication and the strength of the mucus membranes lining the vagina. When Estrogen levels fall and the mucosal lining is weakened and dry, women become more prone to yeast and bacterial infections. That's one reason they become more avoidant of sexual intimacy. A small dose of Estrogen may completely cure this symptom.

Estrogen is also essential for overall skin health, and women with normal Estrogen levels generally have stronger, smoother skin. This is because Estrogen stimulates dermal fibroblasts to produce more and healthier collagen. It also makes the Epidermis retain moisture. Normal Estrogen levels stimulate hair follicles in the scalp and improve both hair quality and growth.

Very high levels of Estrogen can stimulate excessive oil production leading to acne breakouts, while low estrogen levels often cause thinning, wrinkling and textural irregularity of the skin.

The most significant clinical problem associated with Estrogen depletion is Osteoporosis, skeletal bone loss and fractures. The following graph represents a four-year study of spine deterioration in post-menopausal women younger than sixty.

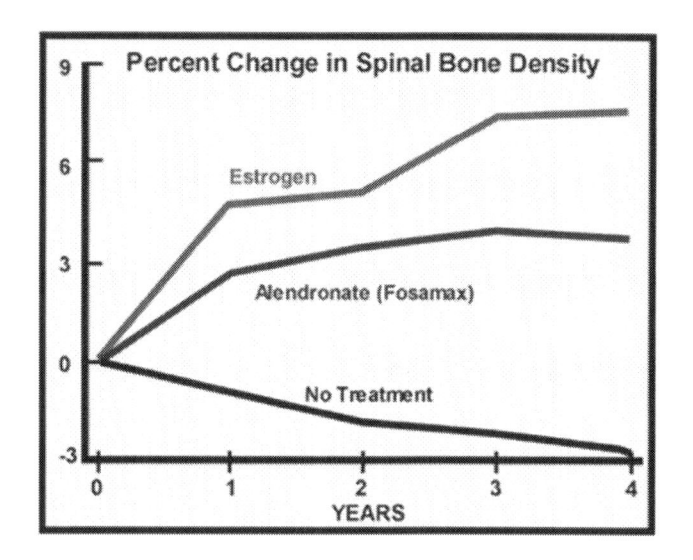

**Percent Change in Spinal Bone Density**

(Graph showing Estrogen, Alendronate (Fosamax), and No Treatment curves over 4 years)

It is clear that Estrogen treatment is a much better option to treat Osteoporosis than the most frequently prescribed medication, Fosamax®, and dramatically better than no treatment at all.

After four years of Estrogen treatment, average improvement in bone density is 8½%. No treatment led to a 3% decline. Even more interesting is that continuous Estrogen treatment, started within five years of menopause, is better than short-term treatment and always better than treatment started after bone degeneration has begun.

We will discuss Osteoporosis and its serious consequences in Chapter 9.

Puberty also brings about a profound increase in female mental capabilities. The reason has only recently been discovered. Apparently the brain has Estrogen Receptors which stimulate the formation of new connections between brain cells or neurons, and these new connections allow the neurons to communicate faster and better. Estrogen helps build the entire neural network instead of just connecting a single wire.

Girls' brains develop earlier and faster than boys' brains - no surprise there - and girls' adult personalities often mature earlier, too. When Estrogen levels fall, up to 15% of menopausal women will experience depression and mood swings. The easy fix, and too often kneejerk reaction of many practitioners, is to prescribe antidepressants. These drugs sometimes work, but are not a reasonable long-term solution. The correct clinical response to a woman of menopausal age experiencing the onset of depression is a complete hormone evaluation and appropriate HRT. Estrogen is essential for a healthy, happy brain.

Ongoing studies reveal that Estrogen replacement, while not a cure for Alzheimer's disease, can slow the process of cognitive deterioration. Alzheimer's destroys the pathways used to store new memories. Without the ability to store new information, everything we've just said, done or seen is lost as though it never happened. It may be that the increase in brain cell connections stimulated by Estrogen forms alternative pathways, a detour that allows new information to bypass damaged areas of the brain.

## The Downside of Estrogen:
## Breast Disease and Blood Clots

There are undeniable links between Estrogen and breast cancer in women with first degree relatives who have had the disease. The risk can be minimized by testing for the "breast cancer gene" and by using a little Progesterone in combination therapy. Nonetheless, the conscientious practitioner should not prescribe Estrogen HRT to women with any history of breast cancer in her immediate family, or to women with a history of any form of breast disease.

Progesterone decreases the effect of Estrogen on breast tissue and therefore, decreases the likelihood of fibrous cysts, as well as benign and malignant tumors. Combination therapy with Bio-Identical Estrogen in combination with Progesterone is preferable to Estrogen therapy alone.

It's important to know that virtually all studies linking Estrogen to breast cancer were based on women using *synthetic* hormone compounds. It is unfortunate that no significant study has been performed attempting to link *bio-identical* Estrogen to breast disease or to compare bio-identical to synthetic hormone replacement.

Estrogen plays an essential role in normal blood clotting by stimulating the liver to produce some of the proteins responsible for forming clots. Synthetic Estrogens taken in pill form, such as birth control pills, pass from the digestive tract directly into the liver without entering the blood stream first. Synthetic Estrogen-like compounds are substantially stronger than bio-identical hormones and cause a significant increase in the risk of dangerous clot formation. The effect of Synthetic Estrogen on the liver is faster and much stronger than the effect of topical creams because Estrogen absorbed from creams enters the blood stream first, and then reaches the liver in a diluted, safer level.

Still, I choose to err on the side of caution and do not prescribe Estrogen, even in topical creams, to women with a history of abnormal blood clots. Future studies may demonstrate topical hormone creams do not pose a statistically significant risk of clots. Until that time, however, even topical Estrogen should not be prescribed to women with any history of clotting disorders.

## Progesterone

Progesterone is the other "female hormone" produced by the ovaries. Progesterone levels rise during the second half of the menstrual cycle because, if pregnancy occurs, Progesterone alters the lining of the uterus to provide nutrition for the developing embryo. Progesterone levels continue to rise throughout pregnancy to keep the uterine lining thick, healthy, and able to fight off cells that could damage the placenta. It also stimulates the growth of breast tissue just as it does during puberty.

Progesterone has a very beneficial effect on the Dermis. It stimulates collagen formation and decreases collagen destruction, a double effect which is lost after menopause without Progesterone Replacement Therapy.

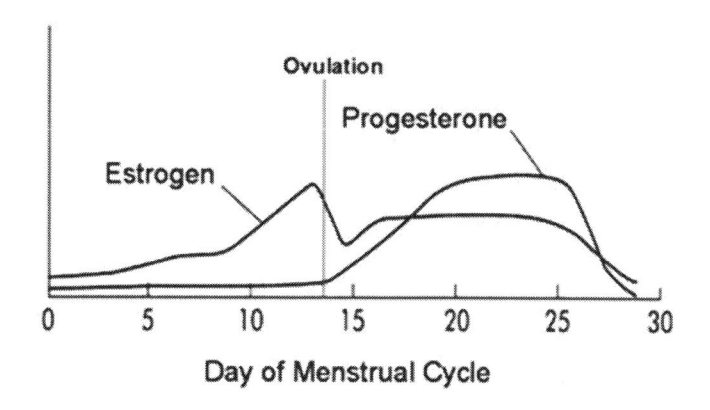

*Day of Menstrual Cycle*

Menopausal woman secrete lower levels of both Estrogen and Progesterone and, therefore, have spotty or irregular periods. Renewing the lining of the uterus is important, and proven to help prevent the development of uterine cancer. Women who lack protective Progesterone or are prescribed only Estrogen replacement are at greater risk for uterine cancer. This represents another prime example of why combination therapy with bio-identical Estrogen *and* Progesterone is so important.

It may also be that Premenstrual Syndrome (PMS) is related to Progesterone, possibly because one side effect of Progesterone is mild sedation. Estrogen alone without Progesterone can lead to emotional irritability. The exact mechanism of PMS is unclear, but we do know that, when less Progesterone is released, PMS is much more likely to occur.

Most if not all the problems associated with Progesterone Therapy relate to the specific synthetic Progesterone, *Medroxyprogesterone Acetate*. Unfortunately, it is the most commonly prescribed Progesterone replacement, and is marketed as Provera®, Amen®, Cycrin®. This drug has been shown to increase the risk of heart attacks, stroke, breast cancer, and blood clots. The risk of clots rises even further if the patient smokes.

On the other hand, the risk of these serious side effects with bio-identical Progesterone is diminished because, as noted previously, it is applied topically as a cream, absorbed through the skin, and reaches the liver where clotting factors are formed in a more dilute form.

Despite this fact, Progesterone stimulates breast tissue and should not be prescribed for women with a history of breast cancer.

## Testosterone

The word Testosterone generally evokes images of body builders and action heroes, not sexy women with healthy libidos. However, both images are correct.

Testosterone is the main "Androgenic Hormone," and is responsible for male secondary sexual characteristics such as body hair, facial hair and deeper voice development from thicker vocal cords. Testosterone also builds muscle mass, decreases body fat and increases energy level. Men produce about ten times more Testosterone than women, although women are more sensitive to this hormone, even in tiny amounts.

Women and Testosterone have an interesting relationship. At "normal" or slightly elevated levels, women have more interest in intimacy and sex, are more easily aroused and have more frequent orgasms. They enjoy intercourse more and have more sexual fantasies.

Testosterone decreases body fat and helps increase muscle mass, improves bone density, and increases the sense of well-being and helps lift depression.

Menopause decreases Testosterone along with Estrogen and Progesterone, and proper replacement is really beneficial. Sounds great, doesn't it? However before you run for the door to get a Testosterone prescription, remember that hormones must be carefully monitored and balanced. The correct dose may give you the wonderful results of increased libido and heightened sense of well being. At too high a dose, however, you might also develop a deeper voice, clitoral enlargement and, in extreme cases, a mustache.

All hormone therapy must be based on careful evaluation of lab work and symptoms, and be regularly monitored by a specially trained physician.

## Recap
- The First Law Of Hormone Replacement Therapy: HRT Takes Time. It Is A Process, Not An Event.

- Lower Estrogen levels associated with menopause can cause problems ranging from hot flashes and vaginal dryness to decreased bone density and increased fractures.

- The risks of Estrogen therapy are reduced by using topical bio-identical creams, instead of pills, and combining Estrogen with Progesterone.

- Progesterone renews and stabilizes the lining of the uterus, which has been proven to help prevent uterine cancer. Progesterone also stimulates collagen formation and decreases collagen destruction in the skin.

- *Medroxyprogesterone Acetate*, the most frequently prescribed synthetic Progesterone, increases the risk of heart attack, stroke, breast cancer and blood clots.

- Women with normal Testosterone levels have more interest in sex, are more easily aroused and have more frequent orgasms. Testosterone also decreases body fat, increases muscle mass, improves bone density, and increases the sense of well-being.

# Chapter 6: Sea Salt and Endless Fatigue

While almost everyone knows something about the sex hormones, Thyroid Hormone receives much less attention in the press and therefore, in our consciousness. Usually, only folks who have already been diagnosed with a thyroid problem know about the Thyroid Gland.

That's really too bad because Thyroid Hormone affects just about everything.

The Thyroid Gland naturally slows down as we age. In the prologue to this book, I noted that aging is a chronic degenerative disease, and no organ or system is safe from the ravages of time. Reputable studies place up to 25% of people over age sixty into a group called, "sub-clinically hypothyroid." *Sub-clinically* means bordering on abnormal with no severe symptoms and *hypo* means "low", so *hypothyroid* means lower than normal secretion of Thyroid Hormone.

## Thyroid Hormone
The butterfly shaped Thyroid Gland lies in the front of the neck under the Adam's apple.

Unless the gland is swollen or has areas of tumor-like enlargements, it is difficult to feel at all. In fact, rather than saying simply "Normal Thyroid" during physical exam, physicians customarily write, "No Thyroid swelling or nodules noted." We express the absence of a problem rather than the presence of normalcy.

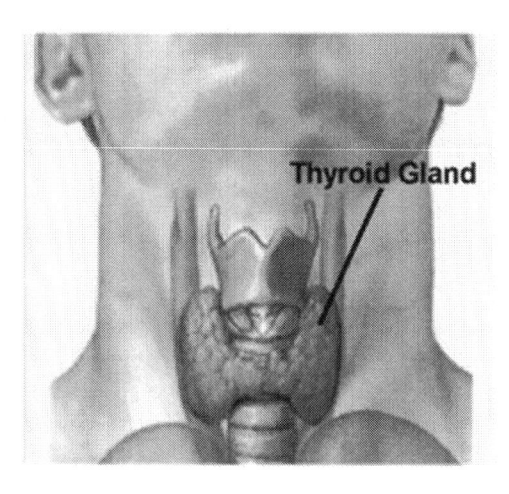

There are two primary Thyroid Hormones: T4 (thyroxine) and T3 (*tri-iodo*thyronine). T3 is a much stronger hormone than T4.

| T3 - Strong Thyroid Hormone | T4 - Weak Thyroid Hormone |
|---|---|
| 20% of Thyroid Hormone | 80% of Thyroid Hormone |
| Created from T4 When Needed; Not Stored in Significant Amounts | Converted to T3 in the Liver Stored in Thyroid Gland and Blood |
| Recently Prescribed as T3/T4 Combo | Most Prescribed Thyroid Hormone |

The Pituitary, a small gland in the brain, secretes a hormone called Thyroid Stimulating Hormone (TSH) which stimulates the Thyroid to produce T3 and T4. Low levels of T4 cause the brain to secrete TSH. T4 is more stable than T3 and usually present in larger amounts. This makes T4 a more consistent marker for TSH secretion by the Pituitary.

If the Thyroid Gland is in good working condition, TSH secretion stimulates the Thyroid to increase the production of Thyroid Hormone. Then, when T4 levels return to normal, TSH production stops until T4 drops again which starts the cycle anew. This is called a *feedback loop*.

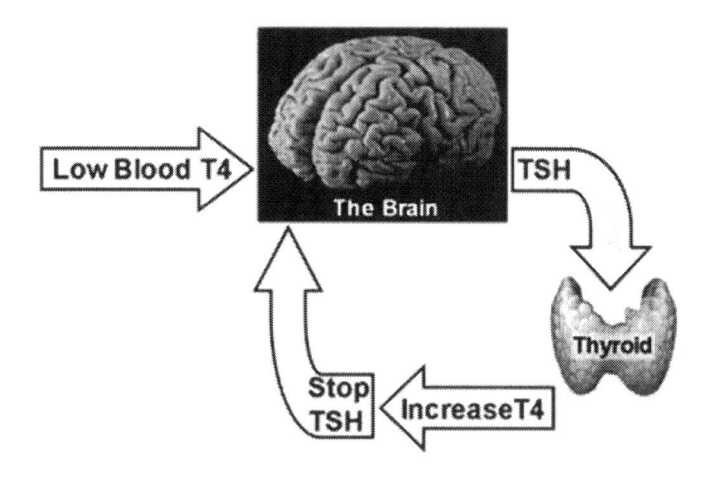

Symptoms of low thyroid include the following:

- Chronic Fatigue
- Unexplained Weight Gain
- Progressive Weakness and Sluggishness
- Increased Sensitivity to Cold
- Coarse, Dry Skin & Brittle Hair
- Depression

Everyone had a grandmother who roamed the house in a sweater complaining of the cold. Chances are, she was suffering from undiagnosed hypothyroidism. It's that common and, in the absence of severe symptoms, frequently undiagnosed.

When a physician suspects a patient may be hypothyroid, he/she may order blood tests for TSH and T4. When the physician finds a High TSH/Low T4 (the brain sends out TSH, but not enough T4 is produced), it usually indicates a hypothyroid condition.

Low TSH/Normal T4 (the brain has stopped sending TSH because there's enough T4) generally indicates normal Thyroid activity. This still does not address the problem presented when a patient experiences mild symptoms of hypothyroidism because levels of T3, not T4, are insufficient. The patient may have normal T4 and still lack enough T3 to function normally.

There are several excellent tests to more completely evaluate this problem. One is called the "Thyroid Cascade Test". By testing TSH, T4, T3 and Anti-TPO (Thyroid Peroxidase), in that order, we can establish where things go wrong during the process of Thyroid Hormone production.

Anti-TPO is a new term worth explaining. In the simplest terms, Thyroid Peroxidase is necessary to attach iodine molecules to thyroid hormone. Anti-TPO is exactly what it sounds like: it destroys TPO, slowing or stopping the Iodine attachment process.

As we learn more about hypothyroid disease and the Thyroid Cascade, more and more physicians are prescribing T3/T4 combinations rather than the more traditional T4, alone. It is my belief this approach addresses the problem more thoroughly; however we cannot be certain until we develop a slow release, consistent T3 supplement.

We're at a point where I can better explain why I "Sea Salt" appears in this chapter's heading? Iodine, the same stuff mom painted on cuts and scrapes, is essential for normal thyroid function. TPO attaches Iodine molecules to Thyroid Hormone. Dietary consumption is the only way we get Iodine and, unfortunately, it is found in very few foods.

In the early 1920s it was recognized that people in certain geographic areas consumed very little Iodine and had more Goiter, the visible swelling of the Thyroid Gland in the neck, and likewise, more hypothyroid disease. In contrast, in places like Japan where kelp (seaweed) is a significant part of the diet, there was very little hypothyroid disease.

Seaweed contains relatively high amounts of Iodine. An easy solution to this problem was to *iodize* salt, since extremely small amounts of Iodine are sufficient and almost everyone uses some table salt every day.

Then, in the 1980s, "salt" became a dirty word. The medical community may move at a snail's pace, but consumers are extremely susceptible to misinformation and medical fads. We frequently make sweeping dietary changes fueled only by media hype and pseudo-science. (Remember when the media convinced us sugar caused hyperactive kids? Now we know it causes **fat** kids.)

Salt became synonymous with high blood pressure and everyone in earshot lowered their salt consumption – and unfortunately their consumption of the essential Iodine contained in iodized table salt. No one seemed interested in the facts.

The facts are these: if you are African American, have high blood pressure, are over 60 years old, or your kidneys don't work, then salt *is* a real problem. If you do not fall into any of these groups, salt can only hurt you the way the Bible says God punished Lot's wife: He got angry and transformed her into a pillar of salt. (Non-believers think Lot's wife ate too many salty giant pretzels at the megamall in Sodom.)

The next Iodine disaster came in the form of a "chic attack." Sea salt became all the rage, first at posh restaurants and then in our homes. Yes, salt derived from sea water tastes more complex and interesting than traditionally mined table salt, but it also contains less Iodine.

It is not necessary to take Iodine supplements. After all, the required daily intake is *extremely* small; 150 micrograms (5/*millionths* of an ounce). Instead, most people should simply resume consumption of iodized table salt, adding some kelp to your diet, and seeing your physician if you feel sluggish, fatigued, gain weight without increasing your caloric intake, or feel colder than the people around you.

## Recap

- The Thyroid Gland naturally slows down as we age. Up to 25% of people over sixty are hypothyroid or sub-clinically hypothyroid, and would benefit from Thyroid Hormone Replacement therapy.

- Symptoms of hypothyroid disease include chronic fatigue, unexplained weight gain, progressive weakness and sluggishness, increased sensitivity to cold, coarse dry skin and brittle hair, and depression.

- A lab test called the Thyroid cascade will systematically test TSH, T4, T3 and Anti-TPO to discover where thyroid hormone production fails.

- While traditional hypothyroid treatment prescribes T4, alone, treatment with both T3 & T4 is probably better. Further studies are needed.

- Iodine is absolutely essential for proper Thyroid function. The best sources of dietary Iodine are iodized salt, kelp and other types of seaweed.

# Chapter 7: You're Stressing Me Out!

## Chronic Fatigue

You've gone from physician to physician, complaining of chronic fatigue, difficulty concentrating and a general feeling of malaise. Your sex drive is low, you can't sleep and you're always sniffling and sneezing. The doctor ordered a slew of blood tests, all of which came back "normal," and told you to "get more sleep" or "take a vacation."

Unsatisfied with this unhelpful response, you made the rounds of local "alternative practitioners." They might have tested you for Lyme Disease and/or Epstein Barr Virus (the two most unfairly maligned infections in the known universe) and, even if the tests came back "negative" or "equivocal," prescribed mega doses of vitamins, the antibiotic doxycyclin if they suspected Lyme Disease, and likewise, told you to "get more sleep."

Frustrated, you return to your primary care physician. He/she doesn't believe that Chronic Fatigue Syndrome actually exists and proclaims in that serious, all-knowing manner employed by doctors, "It's all in your head. I recommend you see Dr. Shrink for a psychiatric consultation."

Rubbish. You are *not* a hypochondriac. You've just exhausted your Adrenal reserves.

"Adrenal reserves, what are those?"

## Adrenalin and Cortisol

Good question, especially since the exhausted Adrenal glands (there are two, one on each side) weigh only 5 grams each (about 1/6$^{th}$ of an ounce). One sits atop each kidney, so they are also called Suprarenal Glands (*supra* or above and *renal* or kidney), where they are totally ignored until you (and they) are almost too tired to care anymore.

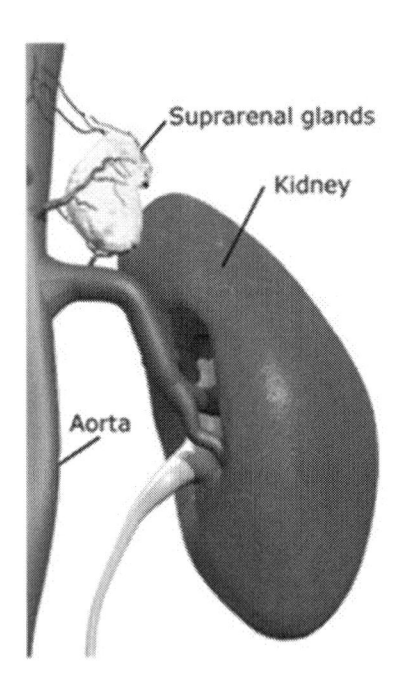

The Adrenals are the "fight or flight" glands. The two most important substances they produce are the hormones Adrenaline and Cortisol. Adrenalin is secreted in response to danger, pain or other startling event. When we're stressed out or in danger, what do we really need? More oxygen is essential in the face of danger. Adrenalin dilates the airways, increases the breathing rate and sends more oxygen to the lungs.

A sharp mind is definitely helpful to combat danger. During a stressful or dangerous event, Adrenalin suppresses areas of the brain affecting short-term memory and concentration. We not only react much more quickly and make better decisions whether to fight or flee; Adrenalin also helps us imprint long term memories of danger. This insures that we're better prepared to confront or avoid the same danger the next time.

Increased muscle strength is needed in times of danger, too. Adrenalin increases immediate muscle strength by forcing blood and oxygen into the muscles. We've all heard about the ninety pound grandma who lifted an automobile off of her grandchild. That's the power of Adrenalin at work.

Cortisol, the other significant Adrenal secretion, provides similar benefits in stressful situations. It improves the efficiency of glucose usage, and thereby triggers a quick burst of energy. Like Adrenalin, Cortisol heightens memory and lowers our sensitivity to pain so we can focus on the stressor or danger and not be distracted by the immediate pain.

While Cortisol and Adrenalin are essential for our response to danger, after the danger passes, it important our body's Relaxation Response be activated. The Relaxation Response returns the body's functions -- respiration, blood pressure, metabolism and muscle relaxation -- to normal. We may feel so drained by the effects of the "fight or flight" response that the resulting Relaxation Response is a welcomed change. It is marked by the deep sigh of relief and the thought, "Whoa! I'm glad that's over."

You may ask yourself, "OK, I was stressed out and in danger, but it's over. Why do I still feel so worn out and exhausted?"

In the ancient world, even in the last century, we lived much simpler lives. We had more manual tasks to perform, but we dealt with them sequentially. There were dishes to wash (no dishwashers back then), meals to cook, clothing to sew, water to carry, etc. The tribe's daily chores were organized and divided among tribesmen and women, and they dealt with only one chore at a time.

Our ancestors never experienced traffic jams, computer crashes, lines at the supermarket, fear that Junior would be late to soccer practice or his Chinese lessons. There were no "urgent deadlines" in day-to-day life. Back then, danger came and danger passed.

In our world, however, the watchword is "multi-tasking," and our poor Adrenals never get the chance to recover from one stressor to the next. No sooner has one passed that another stressor comes fast on its heels. In modern life, stressors just keep coming at us, and it takes a huge toll on our ability to function. As a result, we are chronically fatigued.

No, you are *not* a hypochondriac and you are not alone. The notion of Adrenal Fatigue is highly controversial in medicine. Some authorities discount its significance, but others estimate that up to 80% of adults experience Adrenal Fatigue at some point in their complex lives.

Which begs the question, "What can we do to recover?"

In part, your doctors were correct. You need more sleep. The Centers for Disease Control in Atlanta estimates that 50-70 Million Americans suffer from chronic sleep loss and sleeping disorders, and 35% of all adults get less than seven hours of continuous sleep a night.

Deep sleep provides the perfect environment for healing not available during waking hours. Try to get to bed an hour earlier and, if possible, sleep in an hour later.

## Eight Vital Hours

While you're asleep, your body has nothing to do – except heal itself.

Everyday life is hard on both mind and body. We all suffer unavoidable physical injuries daily, like pressure on our joints and spine with every step, smog and second hand smoke invading our lungs with each breath, just to mention two.

Mentally, we're bombarded with more sound bites and information bytes, and essential and useless communication in one day than our ancestors received in years – possibly, in a lifetime.

Sleeping enough – eight hours a night, *minimum* – and we have time to repair the damage done by just being alive. Conversely, lack of sleep accelerates aging; they don't call it "beauty sleep" for nothing.

Unfortunately, we sleep less today than we did even a few decades ago. The average daily sleep hours has consistently decreased since the 1960s. In 1960 a survey of a million people reported that they slept 8-9 hours a night. Recent similar surveys by the National Sleep Foundation showed the average person sleeps only about seven hours a night. The cause of this change may be debatable, but the effect is crystal clear: we're usually exhausted.

## Sleep vs. Hormones
Vital hormones, including HGH and Testosterone, are produced primarily while we sleep. When we get less than seven hours, production of these vital hormones drops significantly, and in turn, this negatively affects healing and rebuilding muscle, bone and cartilage.

Lack of sleep also affects the production of Cortisol and increases our sensitivity to stress. This, in part, explains why chronic sleep deprivation decreases cell sensitivity to insulin and increases the rate of type II diabetes.

## Sleep and Stay Thin
Sleep deprivation can also lead to weight gain. Although this observation was made several years ago, we have just begun to understand the mechanism of sleep deprivation and obesity. It seems illogical; if we are awake longer don't

we burn more calories? Perhaps, but the problem seems, once again, to be hormonal.

During sleep our bodies produce Leptin, the appetite suppressing hormone. Less sleep - less Leptin – more appetite. Insufficient sleep also makes us produce excess amounts of another interesting substance, Ghrelin (pronounced "gray-lin.") Ghrelin is made in the stomach and stimulates appetite. Lack of sleep creates a double whammy: appetite is increased by stimulation from excess Ghrelin and lack of appetite suppressing Leptin.

## Sleep Refreshes Skin
Most of us are aware that we begin to look pale and worn down if we chronically lose sleep. Who hasn't been told, "You look tired," after a sleepless night? The hormones Cortisol and Insulin only reach collagen stimulating levels during sleep. That's why less sleep means more wrinkles.

## The Dracula Hormone
Melatonin has become a popular over-the-counter sleep aid. This crucial hormone, produced in the brain in response to darkness, really does put us to sleep. Because it only comes out at night, Melatonin is sometimes called "the Dracula hormone" and explains why we tend to sleep better in very dark rooms.

When we're exposed to lots of bright light during in the day, we produce even more Melatonin at night. Insufficient melatonin and, therefore, insufficient sleep can lead to depression, increased cancer risk and a weakened immune system. That's why melatonin is creeping into mainstream medical research for cancer prevention in night-workers, and as a treatment for Seasonal Affective Disorder (SAD) which affects people who get depressed during the winter when the days are shorter.

The message is clear: make sure you get eight hours or more of sleep every night in a dark room. It's a priority for health and anti-aging. You may need to go to bed earlier than usual, or get up later. Whichever way you choose, make sleep-time as a priority. Just do it.

Vitamin C, discussed at length in the chapter on nutrition, is a wonderful adjunct to stress relief. Not only does Vitamin C reduce the sensation of stress and our anxiety response, it also decreases Cortisol secretion so that the Adrenal Glands can build adequate reserves. I recommend (and take) 4,000 mg a day: 2,000 mg every morning and 2,000 mg at bedtime.

Caffeine stimulates the Adrenals to produce more Adrenalin and more Cortisol. Drink less coffee and never take caffeine stimulants. If you feel the need to ingest caffeine (who doesn't love a good cup of French Roast?) why on Earth would you remove the wonderful aroma, ritual of preparation and pleasurable, slow tasting which accompany the morning coffee experience? Also remember it's called "morning coffee." If you want to insure getting a good night's sleep, avoid coffee and caffeine after noon.

Here's something practically every mother teaches her children: never skip breakfast. A healthy breakfast really does jump start your day. Eating several smaller meals a day is also helpful because it evens out your use of Cortisol, Insulin and Glucose.

Exercise regularly. This point cannot be repeated often enough. Exercise reduces stress, improves body strength so less "fight or flight" response is required when stress rears its ugly head. It also retards the development of osteoporosis. Yoga and meditation are also terrific stress relievers, and clinically proven to reduce Cortisol levels.

Finally, if symptoms of chronic fatigue persist, request an Adrenal Function Test (AFT). By testing Cortisol blood levels at four different times during the day, doctors can more accurately determine if a patient actually has Adrenal Fatigue. If you have documented Adrenal Fatigue Syndrome with accompanying Cortisol depletion, your physician can prescribe Cortisol to correct the problem. Just remember that follow-up blood tests are necessary to balance your Cortisol level and make sure you don't get too much.

## Recap

- If you experience chronic fatigue and difficulty concentrating, you're not a hypochondriac. You may very well have undiagnosed Adrenal Fatigue Syndrome. At some point in our adult lives, some experts estimate 80% of adults will suffer from it.

- The tiny Adrenals are the "fight or flight" glands, and the two most important substances they produce are Adrenalin and Cortisol. Both are secreted in response to stress, danger and pain.

- In the modern world, the watchword is "multi-tasking" and our poor Adrenals never get to recover. The stress just keeps on coming. As a result, we deplete our ability to produce Cortisol, and we become chronically fatigued.

- Lifestyle changes can greatly reduce chronic fatigue. More sleep, less caffeine, more frequent and smaller meals, regular exercise, yoga and meditation all help.

- If the symptoms persist, insist that your doctor orders an Adrenal Function Test (AFT) and prescribes Cortisol when indicated.

- While you're asleep your body has nothing to do except heal itself.

- Inadequate sleep interferes with Testosterone and HGH production, which interferes with healing and rebuilding muscle, bone and cartilage.

- Decreased Cortisol and Insulin lead to appetite increase, Type 2 Diabetes and obesity.

- When we don't get enough sleep, we get a double whammy: increased appetite from appetite-stimulating Ghrelin stimulation and absence of appetite-suppressing Leptin.

- We build collagen while we sleep. Less sleep means more wrinkles.

- Insufficient melatonin from insufficient sleep can lead to depression and increased cancer risk. That's why melatonin is creeping into mainstream medical research.

- Eight or more hours of sleep keeps our minds sharp and may actually help prevent dementia.

# Chapter 8: When Does Growth Stop?

The answer to this question is, unequivocally, "Never." Yet, there is no greater conflict within the medical community than the prescription of Human Growth Hormone (HGH) to adult patients.

Traditional practitioners do not prescribe HGH as a health adjunct.

In some ways, I find this comforting because most practitioners haven't a clue how to properly augment HGH – note I said "augment," not "replace" – and fewer have the time required in their busy practices to conscientiously follow HGH patients over years of treatment. Careful follow-up is essential because excessive dosing can lead to significant side effects like acromegaly (bone growth of the feet, jaw, forehead, etc.) and enlargement of the internal organs.

Unlike Estrogen and Progesterone which plummet like stones during the progression of menopause, HGH declines slowly over a period of years, starting at around age 35-40. We begin to produce about 1.5% less every year. By the time we're sixty, we are usually below 40-50% of the HGH men and women actually need for optimal performance.

The part of the brain which produces HGH will still produce it as long as we live. However, if we receive too much HGH by injection, we can shut down our natural production completely. That would be classified as hormone *replacement* therapy, a bad idea for such an important natural substance.

HGH should never to be used to *replace* your own production of HGH; rather, it is intended to *augment* and add to the natural hormone you already produce. This process is painstaking, laboratory-guided and individualized according to every individual patient's needs.

## The Master Hormone

HGH is often referred to as the master hormone because it affects every system in the human body. Secretion reaches its peak during adolescence, which makes perfect sense because HGH stimulates our bodies to grow and most growth happens between birth and age eighteen. Production of HGH slows consistently after adolescence.

Our bodies continue to produce HGH, usually in short bursts during deep sleep. Peak production occurs at about age twenty. Production may be halved by age forty, and falls to about ten percent by age seventy.

If I had to single out one hormone that can reverse the signs and symptoms of the disease we call "aging," I'd pick HGH every time. The list of HGH effects and benefits is staggering.

HGH decreases body fat, especially in difficult areas such as the tummy, butt, "love handles" and thighs. The master hormone also boosts *spontaneous* increases in muscle mass and even greater muscle growth in response to exercise.

A 1990 study in the *New England Journal of Medicine* reported that men who took HGH injections demonstrated a 9% gain in lean body mass (muscle) and a 14% loss in body fat without *any* increase in exercise or decrease in diet. It seems absurd that, more than two decades later, this promising treatment has not been better studied and developed.

HGH increases your energy level, ability to ward off infection, tissue repair and cell replacement. It improves bone strength and helps reverse Osteoporosis, stimulates re-growth of liver, spleen and kidneys *after* they've been ravaged by age, improves cardiac output after heart attack or heart failure, and measurably improves brain function. Not too shabby for a hormone the traditional medical community refuses to prescribe as a health adjunct, and which many states (although not the federal government) scheduled as an illegal substance to possess without a doctor's prescription.

## Measuring HGH via IGF-1

By now it should be fairly obvious that HGH is extremely important. Unfortunately, HGH only lasts a few moments in the bloodstream and its short life span makes it extremely difficult to measure. HGH is quickly absorbed by the liver and then converted into growth factors of which IGF-1 is the most important. IGF-1, also known as Somatomedin-C, stands for **I**nsulin-like **G**rowth **F**actor 1.

IGF-1 acts as a hormone just like HGH, but it is much easier to measure because it maintains stable, measurable levels in the bloodstream throughout the day. Instead of using the rapidly changing HGH levels to monitor HGH production, IGF-1 levels present a clearer and more accurate way to monitor HGH deficiency and the success of clinical augmentation.

IGF-1 blood levels range from 10-1000 ng/ml (nanograms per milliliter). While that's a huge relative range, it represents a very small amount: 500 ng = 2/100 millionths of an ounce. For our purposes we'll just list the numbers.

The red asterisk beside the 12-15 year old female measurement is a simple reminder that girls start their growth spurt before boys, and therefore, their early IGF-1 measurements generally will be higher.

| IGF-1 Levels (Somatomedin C) |||
| --- | --- | --- |
| Age | Male (ng/ml) | Female (ng/ml) |
| 12 - 15 years | 202-957 | 261-1096 * |
| 16 - 24 years | 182-780 | 182-780 |
| 25 - 39 years | 114-492 | 114-492 |
| 40 - 54 years | 90-360 | 90-360 |
| >55 years | 71-290 | 71-290 |

In all hormone therapy, optimal blood levels occur at around age forty. This seems to be when most age-related hormonal decline begins and signs and symptoms of the disease of aging start to show.

The onset of menopausal symptoms serves as the perfect example. Blood levels of IGF-1 should be maintained at around 250-350 in patients who have been tested and shown to have IGF-1 deficiency and accordingly, HGH deficiency.

Clinically, the results are exciting to see. Patients lose body fat, gain muscle mass and demonstrate noticeable increases in energy levels. They're excited to take on new projects and feel refreshed and renewed. Any physician prescribing HGH can verify these results; the question is, "How do we achieve maximum results with minimum risk of side effects?"

## Side Effects

Yes, there may be side effects. Any substance as powerful and beneficial, and which affects every system in your body, has the potential for side effects. HGH is no exception.

If your physician is careful to maintain IGF-1 levels between 250- 350, there is very little risk of side effects from HGH therapy. Unfortunately, HGH frequently falls into the wrong hands and that's where the problems usually begin.

Personal trainers, sports coaches and even team physicians have been known to give athletes HGH without any evidence of hormone deficiency. They just want to win games. The athletes take HGH because it makes them faster, stronger and more aggressive. Their goal is increased performance on the field and more money from lucrative contracts, not anti-aging. Greed is a powerful stimulant.

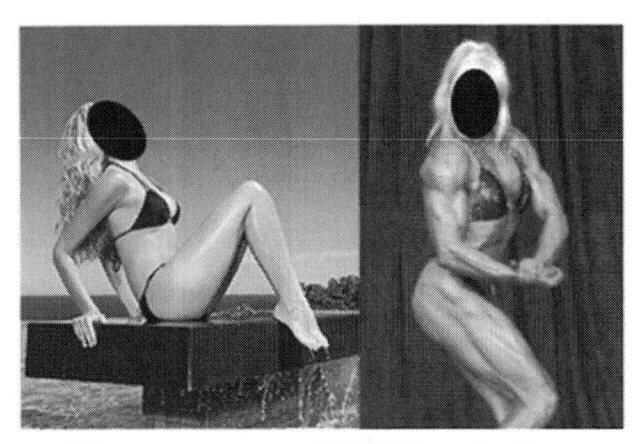

**There are normal HGH levels & ...**

At excessive levels, HGH can lead to carpal tunnel syndrome, a painful disorder caused by narrowing of the nerve passage through the wrist and into the hand. It is most often due to a genetic predisposition because the carpal tunnel is simply smaller in some people. Other causes include injury or problems in the wrist joint, rheumatoid arthritis, work-related stress, repeated use of vibrating hand tools and fluid retention. In excessive doses, HGH can lead to fluid retention and narrow the carpal tunnel.

At high doses, HGH can also cause high blood pressure and even provoke diabetes. HGH has even been thought to increase tumor growth. Certainly, the possibility of existing tumors needs to be addressed before beginning HGH therapy, but there are no studies linking HGH augmentation to *new* tumor growth. Some practitioners recommend a full body positron emission tomography (PET) scan prior to HGH treatment.

PET Scans create computerized images of chemical changes such as increased sugar metabolism. Because tumors have higher metabolic rates than normal tissue, PET Scans can detect tumors of very small size by measuring sugar uptake. I believe this is an expensive and unnecessary step in the HGH augmentation process; tumors should be diagnosed and treated as symptoms present.

The real secret to successful HGH augmentation is careful monitoring of patients' symptoms and blood levels of IGF-1. Practitioners should insist patients repeat IGF-1 levels at three months, six months and one year after initiating treatment. By then, levels are usually stable and yearly re-evaluation is sufficient, barring any episodes of illness or signs which might indicate the HGH level needs immediate adjustment.

## HGH Secretagogues

Charlatanism has existed forever. Whether we called them fakirs, snake oil salesmen, quacks or just plain frauds, their motives were always the same: separate you from your money by selling false cures.

Quackery involving HGH has escalated in proportion to the media attention surrounding its use and misuse. A great number of these frauds sell secretagogues, *i.e.*, substances that cause or stimulate another substance to be secreted.

The Internet is rife with advertisements touting substances taken orally which supposedly stimulate HGH secretion by the pituitary gland. It's all hogwash.

Hence, remember the Second Law Of Hormone Therapy: HGH Secretagogues Do Not Work as Promised and Are a Complete Waste of Money.

Every one of these products -- pills, sprays and powders, "HGH releasers", "stimulators" or "activators" -- bear the following statement somewhere on the label: "These statements have not been evaluated by the FDA. This product is not intended to diagnose, treat, cure, or prevent any disease." 'Nuff said.

## Recap

- Human Growth Hormone is the most powerful and effective protective hormone against the disease of aging.

- HGH declines slowly, starting at around age 35-40. By age sixty, we are usually below 40-50% of the HGH we actually need for optimal performance.

- HGH should never be used to *replace* your own HGH production; rather, it is intended to *augment* and add to the natural hormone your body already produces.

- HGH increases muscle and decreases body fat, strengthens bone, stimulates repair of all vital organs, improves cardiac output and measurably improves brain function.

- The best clinical indicator of HGH deficiency is IGF-1 because, unlike HGH which disappears rapidly, it maintains stable levels in the bloodstream throughout the day.

- In excess, HGH has serious side effects, among them, acromegaly, high blood pressure, diabetes and carpal tunnel syndrome. Most side effects are the result of poor (or no) medical management.

- The Second Law Of Hormone Therapy: HGH Secretagogues Do Not Work as Promised and Are a Complete Waste of Money.

# Chapter 9: She Broke Her Hip and Fell Down

Wait. Shouldn't that be, "She fell down and broke her hip"?

No.

## Osteoporosis

Osteoporosis (from the Latin for "porous bone") is thinning and weakening of bone structure because calcium, the mineral responsible for bone strength, is lost and does not re-deposit in the bones. As a result, bones develop empty spaces called pores and tunnels. Where there was once strong calcium, now there's just air. The photo below dramatically demonstrates calcium loss and serious bone weakening in Osteoporosis.

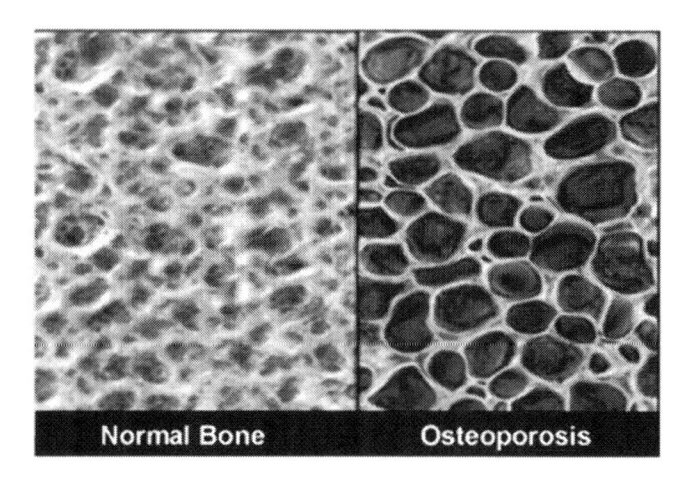

Women are three times as likely as men to lose bone density; dense bone is strong bone and contains a lot of calcium. Thin white women are more likely to develop

Osteoporosis than any other patient group. Men lose bone density relatively slowly as they age, and African Americans, on average, have denser bones to begin with. In the U.S., about a third of all women over fifty have osteoporosis.

We think of bones as stable blocks of calcium, but in fact they are constantly being re-formed and remodeled. The body continuously breaks down bone and releases calcium in it, and at the same time, new bone is being formed to replace it. This balance between resorption and re-formation of bone is affected by several things. Hormones, diet and exercise are especially important, and we can influence all of them.

As women reach menopause, they lose bone-protective Estrogen and suffer marked decreases in both Testosterone and HGH, two other vital bone-building hormones. The resorption/re-formation balance is shifted. Resorption continues and bones lose calcium, but bone formation slows down to a crawl. As a result, untreated women can lose 25-30% of their bone density in the first five years after menopause. After that, the process continues more slowly as a normal part of bone aging, so the bones of elderly women can become very fragile.

To make matters worse, most women don't like to exercise with free weights or dumbbells (not to be confused with husbands or boyfriends). Free weights work both fast and slow twitch muscles to build a stronger, more defined and coordinated muscle mass, and increase bone density faster than any other form of exercise. Any form of exercise with weights will stimulate the re-formation phase of bone remodeling. Resistance exercise may include using rubber or elastic resistance bands or simply working against gravity. The National Osteoporosis Foundation website features specific bone-building exercises.

The third important factor leading to osteoporosis is that women, especially young women, generally consume less Vitamin D and Calcium than needed to preserve bone density. Calcium is necessary to form bone; Vitamin D helps the absorption of calcium into the blood stream and regulates the proportion of calcium, protein and other minerals in bone development.

The recommended guidelines are readily available: before age fifty, women need 1,000 mg of calcium and 400-800 International Units (IU) of vitamin D every day. Women older than age fifty need a daily total of 1,200 mg of calcium and 1,000 IU of vitamin D every day.

Most of us know that dairy products contain substantial amounts of calcium, as do certain fish and some green vegetables. More surprising sources of Calcium are tofu and tahini. An excellent list of calcium-rich foods can be found at the International Osteoporosis Foundation website.

Vitamin D is harder to find in the diet, though fish oil, egg yolks and certain mushrooms are rich sources, and Vitamin D is often added to milk and breakfast cereal.

Vitamin D is also produced when skin is exposed to sunlight, although less readily with sunscreen. Because sunscreen is vital to protect skin, taking a daily vitamin supplement is the sensible thing to do.

Osteoporosis probably has its roots in childhood and adolescence, the period when your body does the most bone building. Some think it is largely inherited and women who develop it simply lost out in the genetic lottery at birth. Either way, there are lifestyle changes that will help prevent this particularly dangerous adjunct of aging.

Women reach their peak bone mass at about age eighteen. Therefore, exercise and nutrition early in life are key to prevent bone loss in old age. Maintaining strong bones is another perfect example of "a stitch in time saves nine." Exercise and nutritional habits are imprinted early in life, and failure to comply can lead to tragic consequences later on. If you have a teenage daughter, encourage her to exercise and eat calcium-rich foods or take adequate daily supplements.

Between the ages of 20-80, the average woman loses 1/3 of her pelvic bone density. In fact, half of all women over the age of fifty will break a bone due to Osteoporosis. The risk of a hip fracture from this disease is equal to the risk of breast, ovarian and uterine cancer combined.

Weakened, fragile bones can break from stresses as tiny as a sneeze. Hence, this chapter is titled, "She Broke Her Hip and Fell Down" because that's what actually happens. An elderly woman with Osteoporosis sneezes, coughs, twists her leg getting out of the tub, or any one of a dozen seemingly innocuous events and her severely weakened hip bone suddenly sheers apart from her own weight. Falling down is the result, not the cause, of the fracture.

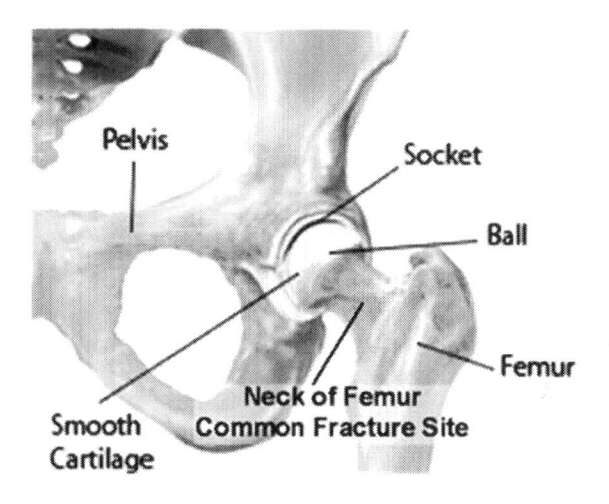

*Pelvis*
*Socket*
*Ball*
*Femur*
*Neck of Femur*
*Common Fracture Site*
*Smooth Cartilage*

The anatomy of the hip joint is very simple. The long thigh bone (the femur) has a thin neck connected to a cartilage covered ball. The ball then fits neatly into a socket in the pelvic bone.

Murphy's Law remains valid: "Anything that can go wrong will go wrong," and usually in the worst possible way and at the worst time. That's why so many women fall down alone at home nowhere near a telephone.

A corollary to Murphy's Law is The First Law of Trauma: The Greatest Stress Always Happens at The Weakest Point.

In this case, the most common fractures occur at the femoral neck, as seen quite clearly in the X-ray below. In the first repair (Case A), the fractured bone was too weak to repair with pins or screws, so an artificial femoral neck and ball (hip replacement) was inserted. Sometimes, the socket on the pelvic side of the joint is also too weak to repair, and an artificial socket must be attached to the pelvic bone (Case B).

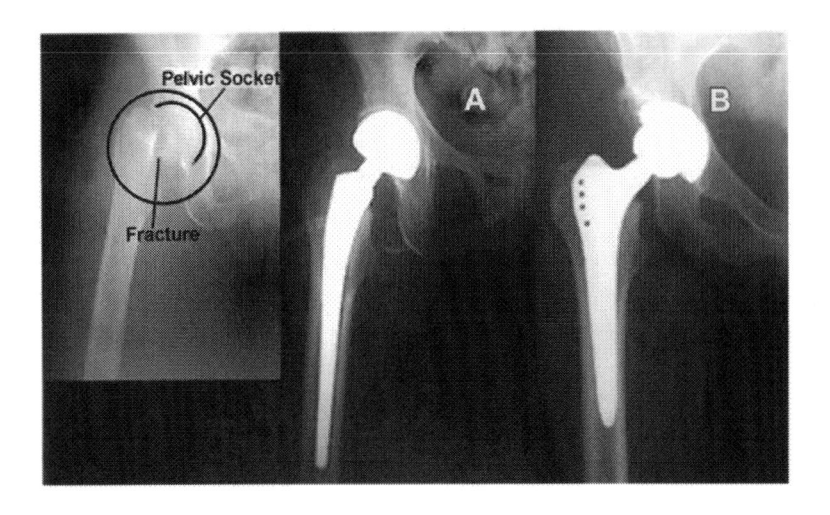

So where does this leave you?

Life expectancy has risen from fifty-three years in 1910 to eighty years in 2010. This increase is directly proportional to clean water, better nutrition, and improved medical and surgical treatments. If our only concern is the length of life, we'd be set. But anti-aging medicine seeks to improve the quality of life, not just its quantity.

We all want those extra twenty-seven years to be quality years in which we continue to be healthy, mobile and strong, rather than years spent in a wheelchair or nursing home bed from which we never arise.

It's not just the hip bones that lose calcium and strength. The spine, arms, wrists -- every part of the body is vulnerable.

We can't stop the clock, we can't prevent most cancers; and we can't stop our hormones from their inevitable age-related decline. We can, however, take the steps described in this chapter which are essential for maintaining healthy, strong, fracture-resistant bones as we age. Osteoporosis may be preventable, but even if it's not, good nutrition and exercise help slow it down. Treat yourself to a great pair of Nike Cross Trainers and, as the ad says, "Just Do It!™"

## Finding and Fixing Weak Bones

If you've already been diagnosed with osteoporosis or if you're over fifty, be reassured that there have been remarkable advances during the last twenty years in the treatment of this disease of aging.

Unfortunately, most women with osteoporosis don't even know they have it. They're symptom-free until they actually sustain a fracture – usually of the hip where so much weight is applied with every step. Rarely, osteoporosis is diagnosed on X-rays ordered to investigate a different injury or disease, but more and more women are getting routine Bone Density studies and most insurance companies now pay for this simple, non-invasive test every two years. They'd rather pay for an inexpensive lab test than expensive hip replacement surgery and long term physical therapy.

All post-menopausal woman, women over the age of sixty-five, and women with a family history of osteoporosis should have their bone density checked regularly.

So what are the appropriate treatments?

Estrogen replacement immediately after menopause will prevent the rapid calcium loss so many women experience. There are certainly pros and cons to hormone replacement therapy, but for susceptible women, a popular regimen now is hormone supplementation for five to ten years after menopause, which is then gradually tapered off. Bones conserve and protect their calcium better if menopause progresses more slowly than Nature planned.

For women already diagnosed with osteoporosis or osteopenia, the weakening of the bone before full osteoporosis develops, there are a number of effective medications available.

Anti-Resorptive medications, as the name suggests, stop excessive bone breakdown, but do not increase bone re-formation. In other words, they halt the progress of osteoporosis. Some of these medications can be taken orally, and others like the widely advertised Boniva™ are given by injection every few months.

A new anabolic drug has been developed which works by directly stimulating the formation of new bone. The best known is Forteo™. This type of drug requires daily injection and is prescribed only for severe osteoporosis.

## Diet Tips

Caffeine decreases the body's ability to absorb dietary calcium. Too much salt or heavy alcohol use will lead to excess loss of calcium in the urine. Cola drinks, which contain phosphoric acid, also cause loss of calcium.

Calcium supplements will be better absorbed when taken with food rather than on an empty stomach. Calcium citrate is usually absorbed better than Calcium carbonate, particularly if taken with antacids like Tums™. Certain foods may be labeled as containing large amounts of calcium, but much of it cannot be absorbed because these foods also contain natural absorption-blocking chemicals. Examples of these foods include spinach, beet greens, beans and wheat bran. If you're worried about insufficient calcium in your diet, consult a certified nutritionist.

## Recap

- Osteoporosis is thinning and weakening of bone structure because calcium, the mineral responsible for bone strength, is lost as we age.

- The First Law of Trauma: The Greatest Stress Always Happens at The Weakest Point.

- Bone formation is complete and reaches its maximum by age eighteen, and exercise and proper nutrition early in life are essential to prevent Osteoporosis when we're old.

- Before age fifty, women need 1,000 mg of calcium and 400-800 International Units of vitamin D every day; after age fifty, they need a daily total of 1,200 mg of calcium and 1,000 IU of vitamin D.

- Hormone Replacement with Estrogen and Hormone Augmentation with HGH reduce the likelihood of developing Osteoporosis.

- Weight bearing exercise, especially with dumbbells, strengthens bones and stimulates calcium deposition.

- Some women should have routine Bone Density Studies.

- Osteoporosis is an enormous problem. Substantial research efforts are yielding effective new treatments all the time.

## Chapter 10: The Body Extreme

The poignant and entertaining film, "The King's Speech" about George VI, reminded viewers that his older brother, Edward VIII, abdicated the throne to marry American socialite and divorcee, Wallis Simpson. This shallow, self-centered, materialistic woman is credited with the popular saying, "No woman can be too rich or too thin."

Okay, "too rich" may apply to women or men, but "too thin" is just wrong. There's a lot more than Osteoporosis at stake.

Being thin without being muscular is as serious a recipe for chronic illness as being morbidly obese. However, the danger of being too thin is more insidious than obesity because, like Wallis Simpson, thin women harbor the illusion that they're healthy because they're thin.

I'm not talking about *anorexia nervosa,* a severe eating disorder characterized by a distorted self-image, refusal to maintain a healthy body weight, an obsessive fear of gaining weight, and a pathological inability to consume food. Instead, I'm talking about anorexia's less dramatic sister disease I have named *pinguis falsus* (Latin for *falsely fat*) characterized only by an obsessive fear of gaining weight. *Pinguis falsus* drives perfectly attractive, sexy women to worry about four or five pounds they gained over the holidays or on vacation.

In general, women are far too self-conscious and self-critical. Their dress feels too tight so they run to the diet doctor. In contrast, men think that they look just fine, no matter how big a gut they're carrying under a baggy tee-shirt.

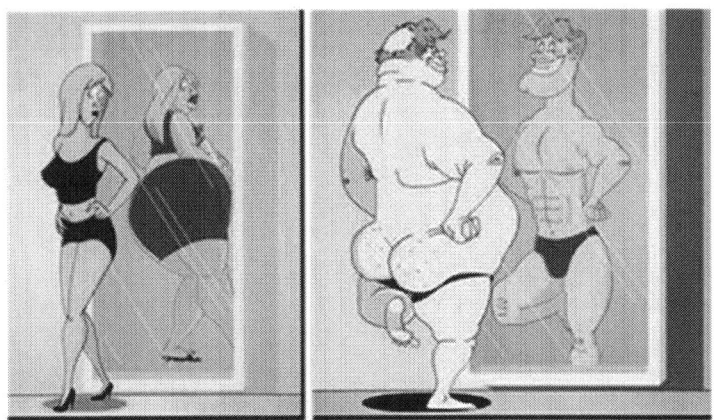

**The Difference Between Women & Men**

The reality is this: no one but a professional prize fighter has a "perfect weight;" the rest of us have an acceptable range of weight. Our weight, within that range, varies day to day, hour to hour.

The first chapter on skin mentions the importance of proper hydration, and our need to drink 10-12 glasses of water a day. Depending on our state of hydration -- whether the bladder and/or bowels are full, how much we're sweating, how much water we've lost in stool production, etc. -- our weight can fluctuate as much as 5½ pounds per day. And none of it is "fat weight;" it's just water.

The lesson to take away from this fact is simple: the scale is your enemy. Never weigh yourself every day; a once a week weigh-in is just fine. When you do weigh yourself, wait until after your daily bowel movement, empty your bladder, and you'll get a more accurate idea of what you weigh.

If you are a few pounds up, cut down your caloric intake for a week or two, add fifteen minutes to your workout, and be patient. It took several weeks of over-eating to gain those extra pounds. Don't panic and starve yourself. In the end, all you'll do is yo-yo up and down ten pounds which is very unhealthy. When you yo-yo diet, even just a few pounds, you lose as much muscle as fat, and drastic dietary changes can lead to unnecessary stress, emotional and even hormonal changes. Worst still, most yo-yo dieters simply return to their weight-gaining habits once the weight comes off, so the cycle becomes endlessly destructive.

I have always relied on a formula I call "The Rule of Proportional Height and Dress Size" as a fair estimate of a woman's appropriate body weight. This dress size provides a better reference point than your scale alone. At appropriate body weight, I recommend the following:

5'0":   Size 0-2;

5'2":   Size 2-4;

5'4":   Size 4-6;

5'6":   Size 6-8.

Yes, at 6'2," that extrapolates to a 14-16 dress size and I assure you a 6'2" woman can handle that with grace and ease.

If you're 100 pounds overweight, you are morbidly obese. You don't need an anti-aging specialist; you need a "lap-band surgeon" and an excellent dietician. All that extra weight you're lugging around carries with it the very real risk of hypertension, stroke, heart failure and diabetes. Lap-band surgery is performed through tiny incisions with virtually no blood loss, but it is still surgery, and has intrinsic risks like all surgeries. Those risks are small, however, compared to the risk of chronic illness and death due to morbid obesity. If you're fortunate enough not to have hypertension, heart failure or diabetes already, the surgical risks decrease further.

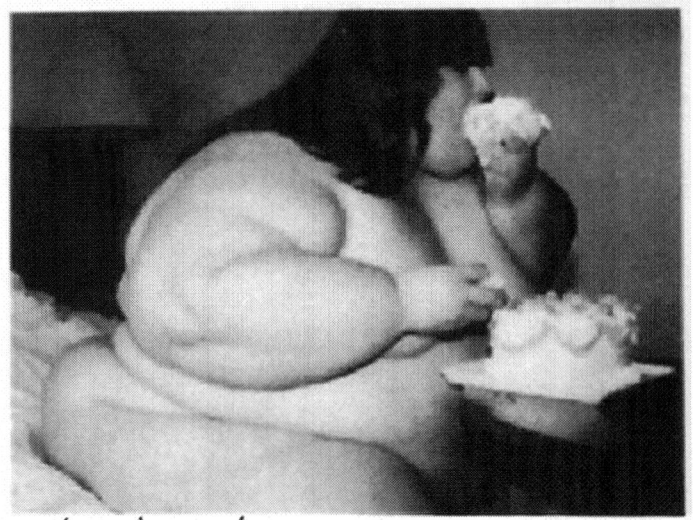

Artist: John Yeadon, Coventry, UK

Don't be fooled by television programs and "fat pride" groups proclaiming that you can be obese and healthy. This is false. Being obese is never healthy. You can be obese without health consequences for while, but in the long term, you're headed for major, chronic health problems. How many morbidly obese seventy year olds do you know? "Healthy obese" is an oxymoron, and those who believe they can be healthy and obese are moronic.

## Prehistoric You

Evolution is an awesomely slow process. A species might manage to make a few significant changes over hundreds of thousands of years, but those changes are almost universally fueled by environmental necessity.

Mankind is the first species that learned how to substantially control the environment; to build shelters, plant crops and cure diseases. This is definitely a good thing, but it comes at a steep evolutionary price; we have virtually extinguished the need to evolve. We are no longer modified as a species by survival of the fittest.

As recently as 20,000 years ago -- a mere nanosecond in evolutionary time - a hunter-gatherer with poor eyesight simply died of starvation. His visual impairment meant he could neither hunt nor gather effectively, much less escape from cave bears and saber tooth tigers, so he died young before he could reproduce and pass along his genes for bad eyesight.

The halt and lame suffered the same cruel fate. As a result, the remainder of our species grew stronger, smarter and better equipped to deal with the vicissitudes of pre-historic life. Back then, a healthy life span was only about twenty years. As cruel as it may sound, we were all too occupied seeking safety, shelter, warmth and food to care about a few weak stragglers.

Modern life means we can eat whatever we want, whenever we want. But our dietary needs remain identical to those of our ancient ancestors.

Imagine, for a moment, what our diet would have looked like 20,000 years ago. Carbohydrates were scarce. Even before the last ice age, we were fortunate to have fruit and grain four or five months a year, as we had no way to store food. Few nomadic hunter-gatherers lugged around refrigerators.

During the few warm months, we gorged on carbohydrates. They were stored as body fat just as they are to this day. All that fat was specifically intended to insure our survival in the lean, cold winter months.

As ice age glaciers moved further south, carbohydrates simply receded into distant memory. What was left on the flat rock which served as our dining table was either meat or fish, both of which required greater effort to secure than fruits and grains.

Hunting with primitive weapons is extremely demanding physically. It involves crawling, climbing and running after prey, and hauling killed game miles back to our waiting, hungry tribe. A hunt could last for days, and we were always hungry. Which begs the question, "How did we survive?"

We survived by converting stored fat back into carbohydrates, thus fueling our hunts and insuring our winter survival. Game meat is protein and fat. It has no carbohydrates. We didn't store it, we metabolized it. Our bodies were engineered over millennia of necessity-driven evolution to selectively metabolize fat and protein over carbohydrates.

We did not sandwich our mastodon or elk between a sesame-seed bun, or slather it with sugar-rich catsup, or enjoy it with a side of French fries. We did not have domesticated animals to provide milk, and no ice cream was on the menu. We did not make club sandwiches with three slices of white bread.

In other words, evolution dictates that a healthy diet is a balanced diet with protein topping the menu. Add in a few fats, especially olive oil and Omega fish oils, and keep your carbohydrate intake to a minimum. It's easy.

How much is enough? A healthy, active adult (as opposed to a slovenly couch potato) requires about 2,000 calories a day. If you are trying to lose weight, drop that number to 1,500 calories and you'll lose about a pound a week. Remember that one pound of fat equals 3,500 calories. If you want to gain weight (rare in these times), add 500 calories a day and you'll gain about a pound a week.

If want to lose weight stored as body fat, the best place to start is by calculating what you're actually eating every day. Do this for a week. It's pretty easy because most foods have nutritional information on the label. There are also many useful, pocket-sized calorie counters available, and websites such as http://www.calorie-charts.net which make the process easier. Here we go.

Day 1 Breakfast

- ✓ 6 oz. unsweetened grapefruit juice, 72 cal, 16 gm carbs;
- ✓ 2 large eggs, 100 cal, 7 gm fat, 6 gm protein;
- ✓ 1 tsp olive oil, 40 cal, 4.5 gm fat;
- ✓ 1 tsp of sugar (in coffee), 15 cal, 3 gm carbs;
- ✓ 1 oz milk (in coffee), 18 cal, 1 gm fat, 1.5 gm carbs, 1 gm protein.

Breakfast: 245 cal / 20.5 carbs / 12.5 gm fat / 7 gm protein.

Do the same calculation for every meal and snack for a week. It will serve at least three important purposes. First, it will make you conscious of what you eat. Most of us have no clue. Second, you'll see where the calories come from; carbs, fat or protein. Third, you can decide where cutting down will be easiest and most effective for you. Be your own diet planner. Empower *yourself*, not Kirstie or Valerie.

Scan and print the following page, or create it with a word processor, and get started.

Every Woman's Guide to Anti-Aging Medicine

| Day: | Date: / / | Target Calories: |  |
|---|---|---|---|
| Meal: | | Grams | |
| Food: | Cal: | Carb: | Fat: | Protein: |
| | | | | |
| TOTAL: | Cal: | Carb: | Fat: | Protein: |

"Target Calories" means the intake goal you hope to achieve, not the actual calories you're currently taking in. Eat as you normally do. Cut down on nothing the first week. That way, when you begin to cut foods and calories, you'll know what you must do to reach that Target Calorie level.

The Day 1 Breakfast chart would look like this:

| Day: 1 | | Date: xx / xx / | | Target Calories: 1500 | |
|---|---|---|---|---|---|
| Meal: Breakfast | | | | Grams | |
| Food: | Cal: | Carb: | Fat: | Protein: |
| Grapefruit Juice | 72 | 16 | | |
| 2 Eggs | 100 | | 7 | 6 |
| Olive Oil 1 Tsp | | 40 | 4.5 | |
| Sugar 1 Tsp | 15 | 3 | | |
| Whole Milk 1 oz | 18 | 1.5 | 1 | 1 |

Drop the grapefruit juice and seventy two calories of carbs disappear in a single meal. Your 245 calorie breakfast just became a healthier 182 calories – 29% less - and you'll hardly even notice the difference. The same 29%, taken away from a full 2,000 calorie diet removes 580 calories a day. Bingo.

## Kick Start Your Diet
Most people believe the first ten pounds are the easiest to lose, and they are right. The first pounds represent mostly water weight instead of stored body fat. There is, however, a way to make the first twenty pounds really count: burn fat selectively and you can lose eighteen pounds or more in six weeks.

"Eighteen pounds in six weeks? I'll be dying of hunger all the time!"

No, you won't, and here's why: you only get very hungry when your blood sugar drops. The process of converting fat into carbohydrates is smooth, stable and continuous. Your blood sugar won't spike or dip significantly, so you won't experience the hunger pangs you have during forced starvation.

People in the diet world like to be called (or call themselves) the "Diet Guru." I've been around long enough to know that true gurus in any field of human endeavor are few and far between. The rest are the pretenders, soon to disappear from our TV screens as fast as they were discovered.

Rarely, we come across true visionaries like Dr. Robert Atkins who certainly deserved the title of Diet Guru. Atkins revolutionized our understanding of the role carbohydrates play in our diet. Had we heeded his sage advice, a third of our children would not be obese today. His approach was controversial, and he suffered constant attacks from the medical establishment, but he was right, and eventually, his ideas were vindicated by medical studies.

Another true Guru was Dr. A.T.W. Simeon, the man who identified the relationship between Human Chorionic Gonadotropin (HCG) and stored fat. In a few words, HCG is produced in very large amounts early in pregnancy to protect the small mass of hormone-secreting cells that maintain the lining of the uterus which in turn keeps pregnancy continuing normally. Pregnant women secrete up to a million units of HCG a day.

In the 1960s, Dr. Simeon observed undernourished women in impoverished countries, despite their emaciated condition, managed to produce babies of practically normal birth weight. How did they do that? Where were those extra calories hiding? He theorized that HCG mobilized whatever tiny amounts of fat these women had managed to store, converted that fat into carbohydrates, and fed it to the fetus. Next, he made a brilliant leap of faith: if HCG released fat for the fetus to metabolize, it might also release stored fat from the obese.

He started to treat obese patients with progressively smaller doses of HCG, and arrived at the perfect dose of between 150-200 IU/day; miniscule when compared to the 1,000,000 IU women secrete during pregnancy, and without significant side effects.

HCG mobilized fat at a continuous, stable level, and 500 calories of food per day was sufficient to provide the remaining energy. Their fat just seemed to melt away.

The protocol Dr. Simeon developed has changed very little in the last decades. It works. When you're only eating 500-700 calories a day, 1,500 calories of stored fat are sustaining you. Over a six week period, you'll burn 63,000 fat calories. At 3,500 calories/pound, that's eighteen pounds.

Losing that first twenty pounds is a fantastic incentive to continue dieting, working with a nutritionist, exercising and improving your self-esteem. I've been on the HCG diet. At age sixty, I felt the scientific evidence linking longevity to normal body weight was overwhelming and decided it was time to drop my excess fat. I lost twenty-five pounds.

You can, too.

Just make certain the physician prescribing the diet will be personally monitoring your progress every week and available to answer your questions. Never purchase HCG in any form on the Internet and never use HCG without a doctor's supervision. Doing so is dangerous. Among other things, improperly administered HCG can affect fertility, alter sex hormone levels, cause acne, depression and increase the risk of ectopic pregnancy.

## All Sugar Is Not Created Equal

For years there has been controversy surrounding which artificial sweetener is safer and better tasting. Every manufacturer marketed its product with a clearly identifiable packet color; pink, yellow and blue. Not one of these so-called "sugar substitutes" tastes at all like sugar and, to make matters worse, they all demonstrate clinically proven ill effects – in rats. Danger to humans has yet to be established, except in the one in ten thousand people with a relatively rare metabolic disease, Phenylketonuria, which is usually diagnosed in the first month of life. If you have PKU, you know it. There is no need to run to your primary care physician and ask to be tested before adding NutraSweet™ to your next cup of coffee.

Food companies got smart and started to experiment with naturally sweet plant extracts; especially Agave and Stevia. This research yielded two sweeteners with no after taste and, apparently, no harmful effects. Many people find they still don't taste like sugar; not even close.

The effect of this sweetener misadventure will be felt by future generations not raised on sugar. Sugar got a bad rap. Consumers believe it has huge caloric value. In fact, it is only fifteen calories per teaspoonful. If you drink two cups of coffee every day, and sweeten them with a teaspoon each, that's a grand total of thirty calories. Remember, it takes 3,500 extra calories to gain a pound of weight. Were those two teaspoons of sugar the only extra calories you consumed a day, you would gain only one pound a year.

It is time to stop blaming sugar in coffee or tea for our weight gain and start blaming other dietary excesses. Eat a healthy, balanced 1,500-2,000 calories a day and you won't have to feel so lousy about enjoying a cup of Joe sweetened the way you like it.

Consumers purchasing sweeteners face a different and more dangerous dilemma: whether to use Sucrose or High Fructose Corn Syrup (HFCS). Sucrose, *i.e.*, table sugar, is extracted directly from sugar cane and sugar beets. HFCS comes from corn.

The United States is not a major sugar producer, so most of our supply is imported. Until the 1970's, our soft drinks and baked goods were sweetened with table sugar. It tasted good and we were happy. Then our government became overly regulatory and, as is usually the case, our elected officials made a mess of things. Congress imposed steep import tariffs on sugar and gave American farmers huge subsidies to produce corn – lots of corn, in fact. Sugar tariffs and corn subsidies essentially forced us to accept HFCS as the principal sweetener in the American diet.

Corn sugar is mostly glucose, the basic unit of all sugars, but it doesn't taste sweet in its natural form. To make it taste sweet, corn sugar must be chemically converted into HFCS with enzymes and heat.

Recently, HFCS manufacturers launched a major television ad campaign assuring the public HFCS is safe. A rugged looking farmer standing beside his John Deere and a field of tall corn proclaims, "Sugar is sugar!" Who could possibly argue with that? I can, for one.

Current research indicates that HFCS decreases longevity in honey bees, mice and rats while the same group of animals fed with table sugar lived longer.

It is not at all certain that honey bees, mice and rats are comparable to humans in this sort of dietary study, but heating corn sugar to produce HFCS leads to formation of several dangerous chemical compounds toxic to both animals and humans. Some react with DNA to cause cancer and others are used to make polyester.

Clearly, none of these compounds should be in the human body by choice. It's small comfort that the FDA continues to monitor trials investigating the risk of HFCS. Such studies generally take years to complete.

The bottom line is this: HFCS is potentially risky. It shortens longevity in several species and is totally unnecessary in our diet. Not all sugar is "just sugar." The safest sugar is derived from natural sugar cane and sugar beets.

## Exercise is Essential

As discussed in the section on nutrition, fat is stored as a readily available fuel source to be used during intense activity. Protein is essential for building muscle. Most carbohydrate-rich foods are essentially useless, other than as a source of fiber.

There are several desirable consequences derived from different forms of exercise; fat burning, muscle building, cardio strengthening and core strengthening.

Core exercises strengthen the core muscles, including your abdominal muscles, low back muscles and the supporting muscles around the pelvic area. They are also called core exercises because they are vital to so many different activities in both sports and daily living. Core muscles maintain posture, balance and stability. Well developed core muscles are not particularly visible. No one flexes core muscles during body building competitions, except abdominal muscles to show off a tight six-pack. That's probably explains why, until recently, the only training which concentrated on core muscle development was yoga. Not surprisingly, yoga practitioners generally stay more flexible, stand straighter and grow older more gracefully than their peers.

> **IMPORTANT:** Before you start an exercise program, visit your physician for a full checkup and make certain that you're healthy enough to work out at your desired level. Always start slowly and progress slowly. Get your doctor's recommendations and do not exceed your safety zone.

Let's begin with cardio-strengthening and fat burning exercise. To burn fat, we need to burn more calories than we ingest. It's simple, really. Subtract the calories you burn from the calories you eat. A sum of zero calories means you will neither lose nor gain weight. At certain levels of cardio exercise, a positive sum (more calories used than eaten) means that you will burn fat.

Your heart is a muscle, and an extremely dependable one at that. It's designed to pump along at a pretty steady rate, seventy-two times a minute, twenty-four hours a day for about eighty years. Most of us, however, manage to destroy our hearts by consuming mountains of junk food and sitting at our desks or in front of the TV for countless hours. A sedentary lifestyle deprives the heart of oxygen and poor nutrition clogs the arteries. Heart attacks don't just happen; we create them.

If you're not genetically predisposed to arterial plaque buildup and eat a healthy, balanced diet, avoiding a heart attack is pretty easy. What follows is a basic exercise guide for a healthy heart and slim body.

Everyone has a range of Target Heart Rates (THR). The range you choose will determine which of several options your exercise session will accomplish. The goal should be to reach your THR during an exercise session and maintain that rate for at least twenty minutes.

It is important not to exceed your Maximum Heart Rate (MHR). There are many formulas, some quite complex, used to calculate this number. I've selected the easiest one available: the "226 Formula." To calculate your MHR, subtract your age from 226.

226 – [your age] = MHR

If you're forty-five years old, your MHR is 226 - 45 = 181.

Next, set a goal for your exercise session, and calculate your THR to arrive at your Healthy Heart Zone and Fitness Zone. The calculations are simple, and you only need to do them once.

1. Healthy Heart Zone -- THR is 50-60% of MHR.
(e.g., at age 45: MHR 181 X (.5 or .6) = THR of 90-108

This is the best zone for people just starting a fitness program. The Healthy Heart Zone decreases body fat, blood pressure and cholesterol. 85% of calories burned in this zone are fats. It also decreases the risk of degenerative disease and has a very low risk of injury.

2. Fitness Zone: 60-70% of MHR
(e.g. at age 45: MHR 181 X (.6 or .7) = THR of 108-127

This zone provides the same benefits as the Healthy Heart Zone, but burns more total calories. The percent of fat calories is still 85% - you just burn more total calories so you lose more fat.

3. Aerobic Endurance Zone: 70 - 80% of MHR
(e.g. at age 45: MHR 181 X (.7 or .8) = THR of 127-145

The Aerobic Endurance Zone improves your cardiovascular and respiratory system and increases the size and strength of your heart. This is the preferred zone if you are training for endurance events such as marathons or triathlons. Only 50% of the calories you burn come from fat, so you must add high glycemic carbs to your training diet.

4. Anaerobic Performance Zone: 80 - 90% of MHR
(e.g. at age 45: 181 X (.8 or .9) = THR of 145-163

In this zone, you consume the highest amount of oxygen and get the maximum cardio-respiratory improvement. Your endurance will improve dramatically and you'll be able to fight fatigue better. This is a high intensity zone which burns more calories, although only 15 % from fat. That's no longer significant because only trained athletes can safely enter this zone, and they are already lean. Olympic swimming champion, Michael Phelps, consumes 10,000 calories per day, much of it from protein and high glycemic carbohydrates.

A heart rate monitor is a great way to keep track of your heart rate while exercising. I personally like the MIO Classic Select, which costs between $35-55 online. It permits you to decide whether you want to lose weight, gain weight, or simply maintain your shape. Key in your personal information - age, gender, weight and resting heart rate – and the device will do the rest.

The MIO Classic Select is worn like a wrist watch and the ample display is clearly visible during your cardio workout.

Without a doubt, the best exercise for reaching any of these Target Heart Rates is running. Our hunter-gatherer ancestors had no other option but to run after their food. Their primitive weapons were only effective at short range. To get a meal, they had to get close to their prey. Because our ancestors only lived about twenty years, the fact that runners inflict constant damage to their knees, hips and ankles never really mattered. They died before joint deterioration and arthritis set in.

Unlike our prehistoric ancestors, we live many decades longer, and need to keep our joints flexible for a life which may exceed the ninety year mark. Impact exercises such as running are too damaging over a long life. A 150-pound runner endures up to ninety tons of force (18,000 pounds) per knee and hip during a one-mile run. He or she endures ninety tons of joint stress in about six minutes. Calculate that out to a 5K race and you're in the 90,000 pounds of damage range. Running for recreation and exercise is self-destructive. The endorphins which give you a "runner's high" will be long forgotten when you're pushing a walker at age seventy.

The obvious question is, "How can I get the wonderful kinetic, calorie-burning, cardio-stimulating, endorphin-releasing benefits of running without destroying my knees and hips in the process?" I recommend the non-impact elliptical trainer to all my patients.

"Ellipticals" as they are called, move in a smooth, natural pattern while your feet stay firmly on the foot boards. No impact and no damage; just gliding along until you reach your exercise Target Heart Rate.

A lifetime of frequent exercise – about thirty minutes a day - is a key difference between a healthy, strong and vibrant you at age eighty instead of a stooped over, home-bound, fracture-in-the-making elderly person. That's why exercise equipment is not the place to scrimp and save. Machines like the **Sole E35 or the** NordicTrack AudioStrider 990 Pro cost in the $1,000 range. If you're serious and plan on using the machine for at least ten years, that's a paltry $100/year.

Fat-burning and cardio achieve the best results when alternated with core and muscle building routines. Do cardio on Monday, Wednesday and Friday, and reserve Tuesday and Thursday for core exercises and weight training. Preserve this (or any) schedule and, after a very short while, daily exercise will become a habit – a welcome and anticipated part of your daily routine.

If you're not into yoga, the best core and flexibility exercise is accomplished on "The Ball." This device offers countless strength and movement options, and serves quite well as a workout bench. Adding balance and stability requirements to strength training is a perfect marriage. The Ball is available in several different diameters because one size does not fit all! Select the proper ball diameter for your height as follows:

| | |
|---|---|
| Under 5': | 45 cm. ball |
| 5' to 5'5": | 55 cm. ball |
| 5'6" to 5'11": | 65 cm. ball |
| 6'+: | 75 cm. ball |

Third, buy some dumbbells. If you have space for a full set, go for it. If space is at a premium, look at nesting weights like the innovative SportBlock™24, a full set of interlocking dumbbells that easily adjusts from 3-24 pounds.

The next illustration shows nine examples of Ball exercises, some with simultaneous dumbbell weight training.

Every Woman's Guide to Anti-Aging Medicine

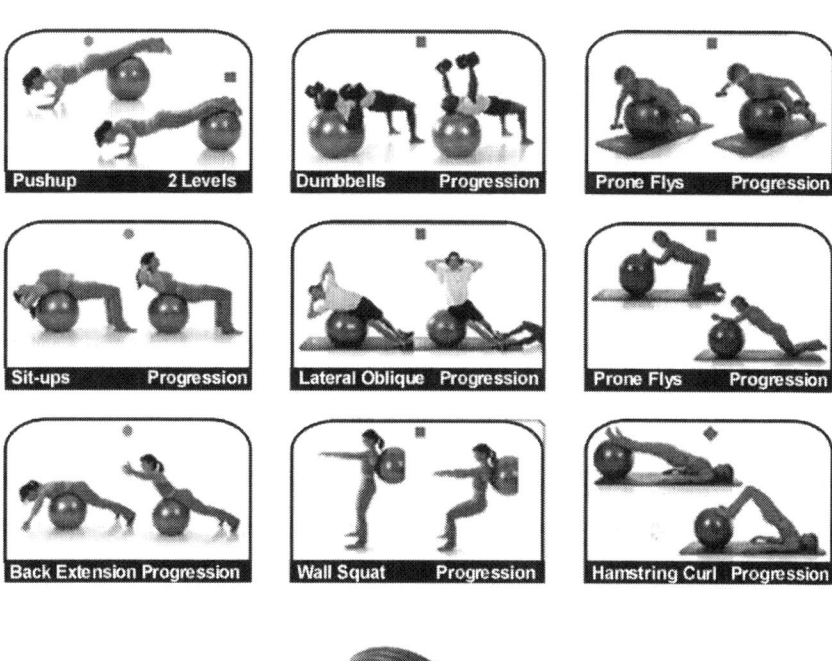

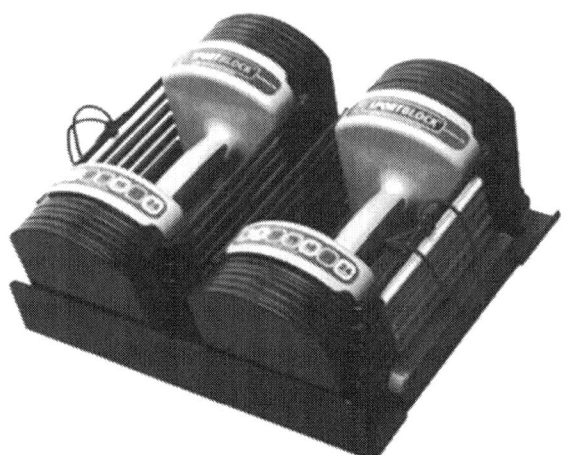

| Pushup | 2 Levels | Dumbbells | Progression | Prone Flys | Progression |
| Sit-ups | Progression | Lateral Oblique | Progression | Prone Flys | Progression |
| Back Extension Progression | Wall Squat | Progression | Hamstring Curl | Progression |

**PowerBlock SportBlock 24**

Using your elliptical trainer will take care of fat burning and cardio. The Ball will strengthen your core. Only weight training will effectively prevent osteoporosis. Besides, strong arms and rounded deltoid muscles can be very sexy.

Remember how amazing Linda Hamilton looked in "Terminator"?

There you have it. Three essential pieces of exercise equipment and they all fit nicely into a small apartment. The $1,200 you just spent bought you an entire gym. Now, use it.

A cautionary word is in order. Don't try to "learn as you go." If you are not a personal trainer, then hire one. In a few sessions, he/she will teach you how to use your new equipment without getting hurt in the process. Doctors see this scenario play out dozens of times: a patient buys excellent equipment, but has no idea how to properly use it. The patient quickly gets injured, never tries again and that fine exercise equipment becomes a dust collector or debuts at the next neighborhood garage sale.

## Bikram Yoga

Yoga is a wonderful alternative to the ball and weights. It has numerous advantages, not the least of which is the constant presence of an instructor and guided levels of expertise.

Bikram Yoga, in particular, is a great place for anyone of any age to start. In a series of twenty-six postures or *asanas*, and two breathing exercises, Bikram provides a challenging, rejuvenating and effective yoga experience. Breathing is especially important because so few of us ever really stretch our ribcage to capacity and maximize our oxygen intake. Each session lasts about ninety minutes, during which you'll work every muscle, tendon, ligament and joint in your body.

Bikram Yoga is practiced in a heated room where, at 95-100°, you'll sweat enough to cleanse your body, and tone muscles and stretch ligaments with far less chance of injury. Stretching and working cold muscles and ligaments is practically a prescription for injury. Whatever your age, weight or prior yoga experience, Bikram will strengthen your body and soothe your mind in ways you never thought possible.

## Vitamins and Minerals on the Cheap

You can buy nutritional supplements anywhere. There's a store on every corner and a website on every screen selling them.

Of the hundreds of supplements available, I present my favorite six, all found at my favorite website, http://www.puritan.com. Not only does Puritan's Pride sell inexpensive, high quality supplements, but occasionally the company has sales of two for the price of one, or even five for the price of two. That's the time to stock up on a year's supply.

1. Green Source®: two bottles of 240 Caplets (480 total) for $57.99. Green Source® is a specialty multivitamin/multimineral with whole food concentrates, antioxidants, Omega 3s, flaxseed, probiotics and digestive enzymes. Because no one can possibly consume enough vital nutrients, even from the healthiest diet, everyone can benefit from a single multi-vitamin taken every day.

2.     Vitamin C – 1,000 mg: five bottles (1,000 capsules) for $43.98. Vitamin C is a great antioxidant. It's essential to countless functions in the body, including production of collagen, and is one of the leading vitamins for immune support. Linus Pauling was a Nobel Laureate, one of the most influential chemists in history, and ranks among the most important scientists of the 20$^{th}$ Century. Dr. Pauling took high daily doses of Vitamin C and died at ninety-three still sharp as a tack.

Pauling's detractors said that most of the Vitamin C we take is simply excreted. Even if that were true, high doses make more Vitamin C available when and if the body is in need. Whether the need arises from a bout of flu or recovery from a strenuous exercise session, you'll be glad you're on a high dose of Vitamin C.

Even conservative medical literature agrees the benefits of vitamin C include prevention of complications during illness, protection against immune system deficiencies, cardiovascular disease, prenatal health problems, eye disease, and even skin wrinkling. Vitamin C assists in faster wound healing the same way it preserves healthy skin; increased collagen production builds stronger scars. High levels of Vitamin C may also be an excellent way to gauge overall nutrition.

3.     Calcium - Vitamin D - Magnesium (1,000 mg - 500 mg - 400 IU): two bottles (480 pills) for $18.99. Calcium is essential to fend off Osteoporosis and build strong bones. Vitamin D is essential for healthy bones, too. Magnesium, along with a host of other benefits, prevents calcium-related

constipation. The U.S. Institute of Medicine of the National Academy of Sciences recommends five micrograms (200 IU) a day for everyone under the age of fifty, and after fifty, increases that recommendation to ten micrograms daily (400 IU). This one, inexpensive tablet has it all.

4.　Omega-3 Fish Oil 1,200 mg: two bottles (400 softgels) for $18.99, and they're purified to eliminate mercury. People with circulatory and clotting problems may benefit from supplements containing EPA and DHA which stimulate blood circulation, increase the breakdown of fibrin (a compound involved in clot formation). Additionally, Omega-3 fish oils have been shown to reduce blood pressure. There is some scientific evidence that regular intake of Omega-3s may reduce the risk of heart attack and prevent cardiac arrhythmias.

Some recent preliminary studies have shown that Omega Oils may slow the progress of rheumatoid arthritis and new evidence indicates that EPA supplementation is helpful in cases of depression and can reduce anxiety.

5.　Glucosamine - Chondroitin - MSM: two bottles (480 capsules) for $37.99. Glucosamine Chondroitin MSM provides support to joints and connective tissues. According to the Mayo Clinic, they ease the pain of osteoarthritis, especially for the knees. This is an important supplement combination for all athletes, beginners and experts alike.

Other clinical trials have shown that glucosamine helps prevent or slow down the loss of joint cartilage. That's another reason why anyone who plans to start an exercise program would do well to consider starting this important supplement combination.

Chondroitin sulfates are synthesized in chondrocytes (cartilage producing cells) and in bone cells, themselves. Chondroitin sulfate exhibits a wide range of biological activities and, from a pharmacological point of view, gradually decreases the clinical symptoms of osteoarthritis. These benefits last long after the end of treatment with chondroitin. It has been reported in recent scientific literature that chondroitin sulfate could have anti-inflammatory benefits and a chondro-protective (cartilage protecting) action by actually modifying the structure of cartilage.

Chondroitin sulfates also increase the thickness of joint fluid and allow the surfaces of joints to move more smoothly.

6. Chromium Picolinate 200 mcg: two bottles (500 tablets) for $7.69. Chromium is a trace mineral and essential nutrient. It's found in the body in very tiny amounts which makes Chromium supplementation especially important. In healthy people chromium functions as a glucose tolerance factor, improving our metabolism of carbohydrates.

As we age, our cells develop insulin resistance - our own insulin is not only released more slowly, but becomes less effective in moving glucose into the cells where it can be utilized. Chromium supplements help reverse that resistance.

Mounting evidence also indicates that chromium picolinate supplementation can lower fasting blood sugar, lower insulin levels and improve insulin usage in people with Type 2 Diabetes, and may decrease weight gain and fat accumulation in patients taking a prescription drug called sulfonylurea, which acts by increasing insulin release from the beta cells in the pancreas.

Higher chromium doses might be more effective and work more quickly. Higher doses may also lower the level of cholesterol and triglycerides in some people. While these findings in no way represent a Type 2 Diabetes cure, it can certainly be considered part of a well constructed overall Type 2 Diabetes treatment plan.

You've just spent $185.63 for at least a year of proper vitamin and mineral supplementation. That's only 51¢/day; an amazingly good deal.

## Recap

• Being thin without being muscular is as much a recipe for chronic illness as being morbidly obese, but more insidious because thin women harbor the illusion they are healthy because they are thin.

• Your scale is your enemy. Never weigh yourself every day; once a week is just fine. Wait until after your daily bowel movement and after you empty your bladder to get a generally accurate measurement.

- The First Rule of Nutrition: A 5' Woman Looks Best as a Size 0-2; 5'2":Size 2-4; 5'4":Size 4-6, etc.

- There is no such thing as "healthy and obese."

- Our bodies were engineered over millennia of necessity-driven evolution to selectively metabolize fat and protein. Our ancestors gorged on carbohydrates which were stored as body fat, just as they are today. A healthy diet is based on protein.

- The HCG protocol Dr. Simeon developed in 1960 has changed very little in the last decades. It works. When you're only eating 500-700 calories a day, 1,500 calories of stored fat sustain you. Over a six-week period, you'll burn 63,000 fat calories. At 3,500 calories/pound, you can lose eighteen pounds.

- There are three essential pieces of exercise equipment: an elliptical trainer, an exercise ball, and a set of free weights or dumbbells.

- The six most vital supplements are: Multivitamin-Multimineral combination; 4,000 mg Vitamin C (half taken in the morning, half at night); 1,200 mg Omega-3 Fish Oil; Calcium 1,000 mg/ Magnesium 500 mg/ Vitamin D 400 IU; Glucosamine/Chondroitin/MSM; and Chromium Picolinate. At about.51¢ a day, it's a healthy bargain.

# Chapter 11: Cosmetic Surgery

If every woman were to start relatively early, and follow the basic plan outlined in the preceding chapters, chances are good she would all arrive at her sixth decade looking pretty darn good.

Firm, collagen-rich skin, stretched tightly across face and body would be the norm. Sun damage and unwanted discoloration would be long forgotten memories, as would be unwanted post-menopausal facial hair.

What, then, would a plastic surgeon do to earn a living?

Most cosmetically unattractive characteristics are correctable with lasers, good healthcare and diet. A few, however, cannot be resolved without resorting to cosmetic surgery. Still, some daring (foolish or greedy) physicians try to stretch the envelope of non-surgical care to the point of ineffectiveness or, worse, danger to their patients. You need to be aware of what lasers and cosmeceuticals can and cannot accomplish.

There is only one reason to correct anything about your face and body for purely aesthetic reasons: whatever you plan to change must bother you greatly. Other peoples' opinions are irrelevant to your decision-making process. That your boyfriend, lover or husband wished you had bigger breasts, for example, should not part of the decision-making process.

Furthermore, every patient must understand that improving her appearance is not a cure for depression, low self esteem or social avoidance. In sum, the decision to have surgery is yours and yours alone, and should be made based purely on personal aesthetic considerations.

All surgery, no matter how minor, carries intrinsic risks: the potential for anesthesia complications; infections and scarring; undesirable cosmetic outcomes.

For one week prior to any surgical procedure, stop taking aspirin, blood thinning medications and supplements. Inform your physician of every medication and supplement you take. You'd be surprised how many seemingly innocuous, over-the-counter pills can cause problems during surgery.

Garlic, Gingko and Ginseng are among the many common supplements which cause poor clotting and excessive bleeding. Strawberries should be avoided the week before surgery because they contain relatively large amounts of salicylates (aspirin). Licorice can increase blood pressure and St. John's Wart can cause prolonged sedation. The list goes on.

## The Eyes Have It

Many women seek treatment for droopy eyelids. Laser treatments should be avoided. Despite statements by laser companies and practitioners to the contrary, lasers are usually ineffective around the eyes. Even the newest laser devices pale in comparison to surgical eyelid correction, or Blepharoplasty. In addition, the heat of any laser device, used so close to the eyes, poses an unacceptable burn risk.

Cosmetic eyelid surgery is a quick (45-90 minute), practically bloodless procedure easily mastered by every cosmetic surgeon, and poses minimal risk to the patient. Better still, the results can be truly dramatic, wiping years from your face.

Blepharoplasty can be safely performed in an office setting under local anesthesia, with or without mild intravenous sedation.

After careful physical and photographic analysis, the incision sites are marked with a surgical pen (usually purple ink), delineating the redundant skin folds. Because injection of anesthetic liquid changes the surrounding contours, marking is always done before local anesthesia is injected. After complete numbing has occurred, tiny incisions are made along the previously drawn lines. Excess skin and bulging fat pads are carefully removed and bleeding, which usually amounts to only a teaspoon or two, is controlled. The incision is then closed with a continuous or "running" suture. The ends of the suture material are taped in place rather than knotted to assure easier removal.

In the recovery room and at home, ice water soaked gauze or soft ice packs are placed over the eyes to minimize swelling and, in some cases, antibiotic ointment is spread over the incision site.

Approximately a week later, the sutures are removed. Over the next 3-4 weeks the tiny scars will practically fade away.

## Nobody Nose

Noses traditionally viewed as "attractive" are not a necessary component of a satisfactory life, any more than full lips, blue eyes or a square jaw. Nonetheless, about 50,000 "nose jobs" are performed in the United States every year.

The line between vanity and the desire to simply "feel prettier" is a thin one. Cosmetic nasal surgery or Rhinoplasty is appropriate for women who desire to improve their looks or functional breathing.

The renowned Danish aristocrat and astronomer, Tycho Brahe, could have benefitted from Rhinoplasty and full nasal reconstruction. In 1566 at age twenty, Brahe lost the bridge of his nose in a duel after an argument about a math problem... a math problem! Instead of surgery, Brahe chose to wear a nasal prosthesis made of silver and gold alloy for the remaining thirty-five years of his extremely productive life.

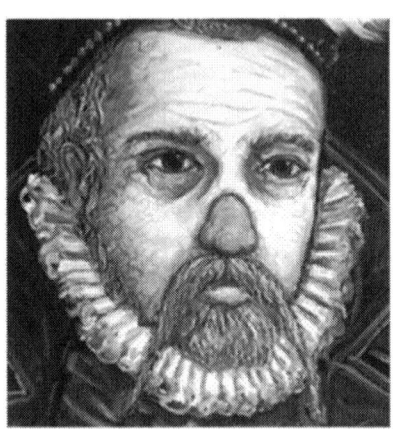

The wildly eccentric thinker also employed a clairvoyant dwarf and kept a pet elk. He reportedly died after a prolonged food orgy which apparently led to massive intestinal obstruction. Some still believe, however, he was murdered to gain access to his tightly protected scientific secrets and discoveries. Gluttony or murder - the jury is still out after 410 years.

As a young man, I broke my nose four times: twice boxing, once playing soccer, and once crashing headlong into the side of a swimming pool after a diving board "misadventure". Fortunately, I had nasal surgery in 1970 and remain quite satisfied with the result.

Unlike Blepharoplasty, however, Rhinoplasty is a complex procedure demanding a surgeon with exceptional skill and impeccable aesthetic sensibility. Nasal surgery should be done by design, not rote, and the resulting nose should fit the face of the specific patient.

Ask your surgeon how many Rhinoplasties he/she has performed. Ask to see before and after pictures of several patients. Do the noses in the photographs fit the faces, or do they all look alike, and seem to fit a cookie-cutter pattern?

Interview several surgeons and then decide. Unless your decision to seek Rhinoplasty is the result of a recently broken nose, you probably haven't liked the way it looks for a long time. Don't allow yourself to be pressured into making a quick decision. Like Tycho Brahe's metal prosthesis, you'll wear your new nose for the rest of your life. Choose your surgeon and your new nose wisely.

## Abreast of the Latest Developments

Breast augmentation is a wonderful thing. Ask any man. In fact, a fascinating 2007 article in *Psychology Today* cited a study explaining the subconscious or, perhaps, genetically programmed reason for this preference. To paraphrase: "...men may prefer women with large breasts because (when the breasts are natural) they have the greatest level of fertility, indicated clinically by their levels of two reproductive hormones, estradiol and progesterone."

Breasts should fit a woman's body like noses fit a face. Few things look more ridiculous than Double D cups on a five foot woman.

You'll know your breasts are the correct size for your body if standard sized clothing which fits your hips and waist properly fills the bust area without being let out at the seams to accommodate your breasts. It's a no-brainer, really. Women who complain that men only look at their breasts while conversing are not good candidates for breast augmentation. The object is to achieve a breast size that compliments your figure; not breasts that draw attention only to your chest.

A full 34C cup bra holds about sixteen ounces or 480 cc (cubic centimeters) of volume, though implants are available from about 125-1,000 (!) cc. A quart is approximately 1,000 cc. Assuming that you naturally have 250 cc breasts, and want to fill a 34C cup, you'll require at least:

480 cc (desired cup size) - 250 cc (your present size) = 230cc implant.

A 34D cup has a volume of 600 cc, and the same math applies: 600cc – 250cc = 350cc implants.

Remember, too, that more that 80% of women have asymmetrical breasts with varying amounts of side to side difference in volume. By properly measuring your present breast volume, your surgeon can correct this difference when he chooses implants for each breast.

One excellent way to arrive at the proper size is to take a dozen Ziploc® bags and fill them, in pairs, with different amounts of rice ranging from 200-500 cc (6-18 ounces). Next, find a lingerie specialty shop near you that correctly fits *brassieres. Don't be shy. A*sk for help selecting a cup size you like, using the rice bags to fill out the cups. Do not go to a department store. Almost 80% of women wear bras which do not fit properly.

Thoroughly discuss your goals with your surgeon. Implants come in different shapes and sizes, and your surgeon will be able to explain the lift, projection and shape that best suites you.

One thing to remember is this: by your seventh or eighth decade, your buttocks and face will sag and your skin will wrinkle. "Tramp Stamp" tattoos and Jessica Rabbit's breasts do not compliment an octogenarian's body.

Over the years, there has been significant controversy surrounding the choice of saline or silicone implants. Original silicone implants frequently leaked silicone into the chest and body, and women developed reactions to it, leading to fibrotic, hard and unattractive breasts and, occasionally, even severe systemic illnesses. These implants were banned and saline implants became the norm.

With the advent of modern, leak-proof silicone implants, silicone has once again received FDA approval. That argument has, for the most part, been put to rest. Silicone feels more natural and the density is closer to actual breast tissue. One additional interesting observation is that saline solution heats and cools faster than silicone gel. In cold weather, women with saline implants tend to feel very cold, and often need to wear additional insulating clothing when skiing or walking in the winter wind.

After the type of implant has been selected, it's time to decide the location of breast implants. This presents another controversy. Some surgeons insist that placement directly below the breast tissue (sub-mammary) is superior and others are equally insistent that implants be positioned below the chest muscles (sub-pectoral). The only apparent advantage of the placing the implant under the breast tissue instead of under the chest muscle seems to be that you get more lift if you want to augment saggy breasts. For every other type of correction, however, sub-pectoral implants yield a superior result for the following reasons:

- Sub-pectoral implants tend to stay in position longer;

- They allow for more accurate mammograms;

- Breasts appear more natural, especially in patients with thin skin; and

- The risk of capsular fibrosis and contracture is substantially lower.

There is no substitute for breast implant surgery. All the ads you see on late-night TV hawking breast enlargement creams and breast enlarging exercise equipment are absolutely and completely false.

## Recap

- There is only one reason to surgically correct something about your face and body: the area you plan to change must bother you greatly.

- Cosmetic surgery is not a cure for depression, low self esteem or social avoidance.

- Cosmetic eyelid surgery is a quick, practically bloodless procedure, posing minimal risk to the patient. Better still; the results can be truly dramatic, wiping years from your face.

- Rhinoplasty is a very complex procedure demanding a surgeon with exceptional skill and impeccable aesthetic sensibility.

- Nasal surgery should be done by design, not rote, and the resulting nose should "fit the face" of the specific patient.

- Studies indicate that men actually prefer women with larger breasts for subconscious or, perhaps, genetically programmed reasons.

- Your breasts are the correct size for your body if they fill the bust area of standard clothing which properly fits your hips and waist.

- For most types of breast augmentation, sub-pectoral silicone implants yield a superior result.

# Chapter 12: Longevity Myths and Facts

"I'll add years to your life!"

The physician who dares to utter these words to any patient is a fool. Undeniably, there are lifestyle choices which can lengthen the average life expectancy, but that's an *average* gain, not necessarily specific to *your* life! Anti-aging medicine is not designed simply to extend life, but extend the time patients can live a *quality life*.

I'm often asked why, having worked in emergency rooms and trauma centers, I still ride motorcycles, climb mountains, SCUBA dive, and bow hunt alone in dense rain forests. It's simple, really. I would much rather die quickly, doing something I love which excites and stimulates my senses, than die of old age looking out from the hospice window wondering what I had missed out on. On a less dramatic note, the same can be said about occasionally indulging in a pint of mint chocolate chip ice cream or scarfing down a two-pound lobster in drawn butter. It's all about balance, not austerity.

We seem to be looking through the glass darkly, so let's take a look at the promises and literature surrounding our length of time on this mortal coil.

## Fitting Into Your Genes

Of all the studies relating specific factors to longevity, those which make the genetic case are the most persuasive scientifically.

Genetic differences explain, in part, why certain families have lots of octogenarians and other families seem to die young. A preponderance of scholarly estimates place 25% of human lifespan variation on genetics; the remaining 75% seems due to environmental exposures, accidents, injuries and chance.

Examination of very long life spans, beyond 90-100 years - appears to have an even stronger genetic basis. Is it equally possible that most long-lived families simply raised more cautious off-spring who looked both ways before crossing the street?

Possibly, but the other side of the equation is more persuasive. Families that tend to die young produce offspring who die young; often of genetically heritable diseases such as certain cancers, heart defects, familial hypertension and the like.

If you come from a long-lived family, lead a careful, healthy life, and don't text while you drive or cross the street against traffic, you get a 25% "leg up" over your genetically less-long-lived peers. If you come from a family fraught with inherited diseases, enjoy the ride while you can.

## Fat Is Definitely Out. Is Thin Really In?

Research findings from the Department of Nutrition at the Harvard School of Public Health and Brigham and Women's Hospital published in 2004 was unequivocal in linking obesity and premature death. This is very bad news in light of the fact that 60% of the American adult population is obese, as are 30% of our children. Among a plethora of accompanying ills, the obese are more likely to suffer hypertension, heart disease, stroke, type 2 diabetes, and spine and joint orthopedic problems.

We're addicted. Fatty, salty food is readily available on every street corner. Who doesn't love those big, thick pretzels, covered in a layer of large-grains salt and drowned in yellow mustard? McDonalds. Burger King. KFC. Fast food rules the culinary world. Healthy food is nowhere in sight. The fruits, vegetables, lean meat and fish we so desperately need are hidden away in supermarkets. Your local supermarket does not have a flashing light or arches over the door proclaiming "Healthy Food Sold Here." When "salmon and salad time" equal "burger and fries time," medical costs will plummet like a stone.

We don't need to reform healthcare. We need to take responsibility for our lives and lifestyles, especially our diets.

Fat is clearly bad, but is being underweight good? One oft-quoted study correlated thinness and long life – in rats. Rats deprived of excess caloric intake while receiving an adequate, nutritionally balanced diet, lived significantly longer than their normal-weight littermates. In other words, thin rats live longer than regular rats.

Not surprisingly, companies hawking diet products and supplements loved this study. But it begs an answer to the obvious question: "Does it apply to humans?" Most responsible biologists and researchers believe the answer is, "Not at all."

The lifespan of a lab rat is short. The Sprague Dawley Rat, a commonly studied breed, may live about three years. Female rats mature fast, reaching reproductive age at 3-4 months. Their life span is thirty-six months, so they reproduce at only 8% of expected lifespan. Their gestation period, for litters of 8-10 young, is about twenty-two days. Before reaching menopause at twenty months, a female rat may produce fifty or more offspring. Hence, the phrase, "They breed like rats!"

Humans reach sexually maturity at about thirteen years, or 17% of lifespan. Our gestational period is nine months and, in industrialized countries, we produce an average of two offspring in a lifetime.

Therefore, it is an absurd leap to correlate rat longevity to humans. Rats, while vital to medical research, are useful as models only where specific cellular damage and repair, such as cancer treatments, are involved. Otherwise, our disparate metabolic needs and life cycles negate much of the nutritional and longevity research in rats.

## Child Bearing and Longevity

Few women decide to have a baby based on longevity impact. Still, it is not unreasonable for women to ask if pregnancy influences life span and aging.

The answer is "yes and no," depending which of the various conflicting studies you choose to believe.

Early studies used historical records and examined long term survival of women against the number of children they bore. Two famous studies used the British Royal Family and a 17$^{th}$ century French Canadian group with an average of seven children per family. Obviously, neither group is representative of a modern family. More recent studies, particularly several from Norway, were poorly designed and almost impossible to interpret.

Until the early-1900s, about one in a hundred women died in childbirth. In many early television westerns, the male protagonist is portrayed as raising his family alone, his wife having died in childbirth of postpartum bleeding or infection. In the popular TV series "Bonanza", Ben Cartwright had three sons, each by a different wife. All three wives had died in childbirth!

Until the 1990's, medicine viewed child-bearing as a "biological cost" to longevity. A baby, including placenta and amniotic fluid, weighs an average of fourteen pounds and the actual body fat weight gain euphemistically referred to as "baby weight" adds another ten pounds. It's pretty clear that pregnant women carry around quite a load, which exposes them to huge stresses on the heart, lungs and joints.

The developing baby also consumes enormous amounts of nutrients from the mother at a time when her hormone levels shift like tidal waves. These consequences of pregnancy can lead to temporary high blood pressure and gestational diabetes. Even in industrialized nations, a small percentage of mothers still die during pregnancy and childbirth.

Most doctors have observed that women are able to bear discomfort and outright pain better than men. Either by genetic or divine design, being able to endure the painful experience of childbirth is likely the explanation for this phenomenon. Rose Kennedy, though a devout Catholic, once quipped, "If men could get pregnant, abortion would be a sacrament".

Yet, nature exacts a cost on women who do not have children, too. For example, pregnancy and breast feeding lower the risk of breast cancer, and women who have had a full-term pregnancy have less risk of ovarian and uterine cancer. Cancer risk actually declines with each full-term pregnancy. Women who naturally (*i.e.*, without in vitro fertilization) had twins or a baby in their late thirties/early forties belong to a special group with an even longer life span.

In the final analysis, only two clear statistics emerge from all the studies. First, mothers of twins live longer than average, particularly mothers of fraternal twins. Second, women who had babies late in their reproductive lives live longest. Cause and effect, especially for the second conclusion, is not at all clear.

It may be that only super healthy women are able to get pregnant late in their reproductive lives. It is also statistically proven that more educated and wealthier women live longer. Is it possible that their higher educational level leads them to seek out better health care, or that more money makes better care available?

The bottom line is this: aging and life span are not, and should not be, a consideration for any young, healthy woman who wants to get pregnant.

## Recap

- Genetics play a significant role in longevity.

- Obesity and premature death are unequivocally linked, a tragic fact because 60% of the population is obese.

- When "salmon and salad time" equal "burger and fries time," medical costs will plummet. We need to take responsibility for our lifestyles, especially diet.

- While thin rats live longer than regular weight rats, this widely cited study probably has no relation to human longevity.

- Pregnancy and child bearing should not be a consideration for women concerned about living long, healthy lives. While considered a "biological cost" in years past, it is not at all clear that child bearing has a negative impact on longevity, and bearing children benefits longevity by lowering the risk of certain degenerative diseases.

# Chapter 13: The Future of Anti-Aging Medicine

In the great Mike Nicol's movie, "The Graduate" (1967), Dustin Hoffman plays Benjamin Braddock, a young man who just finished college. At his graduation party, a family friend named Mr. McGuire corners Benjamin by the pool and has the following supposedly serious conversation in overly hushed tones:

**Mr. McGuire**: I want to say one word to you. *Just one word.*

**Benjamin**: Yes, sir.

**Mr. McGuire**: Are you listening?

**Benjamin**: Yes, I am.

**Mr. McGuire**: *Plastics.*

**Benjamin**: Just how do you mean that, sir?

**Mr. McGuire**: There's a great future in plastics. Think about it. Will you think about it?

**Benjamin**: Yes, I will.

**Mr. McGuire**: Shhhhhh! 'nuff said. That's a deal.

Aside from exceptional acting and wonderful writing, this humorous scene actually gave us a glimpse into the future. Just a few years later the plastics industry rocketed forward and today just about everything we touch is made of plastic.

Anti-Aging Medicine is like that, too. It offers a glimpse into the future of medicine which no other scientific field can match. The watch words -- Embryonic Stem Cells and Telomerase -- are heard at the annual international conventions and read in anti-aging journals. That's where you'll find the "Mr. McGuires" of the Anti-Aging field, and what they're saying is just as prescient and just as real... but first, some historical context.

## A Lesson in History

Spanish American philosopher, essayist and novelist, George Santayana (1863-1952), famously said, "Those who cannot remember the past are condemned to repeat it." Grave historical errors are repeated so often that Santayana's wisdom has become a sad cliché.

One of the most glaring examples relates to medicine.

Dissection is the process of disassembling a body to ascertain its internal structure, function and the relationships of its components. In 1163, the Catholic Church, by the Council of Tours, issued the *Ecclesia Abhorret a Sanguine* which prohibited the practice of human dissection, and in the early 14th century, Pope Boniface VIII forbid the practice of dismembering slain crusaders for return of their bones to their families for burial.

The ban on dissection lasted four hundred years and medical science in Europe was hamstrung. Indeed, European doctors did not even know there *was* a ham string muscle. Advances in medicine and surgery screeched to an abrupt halt.

**Andreas Vesalius Dissection**

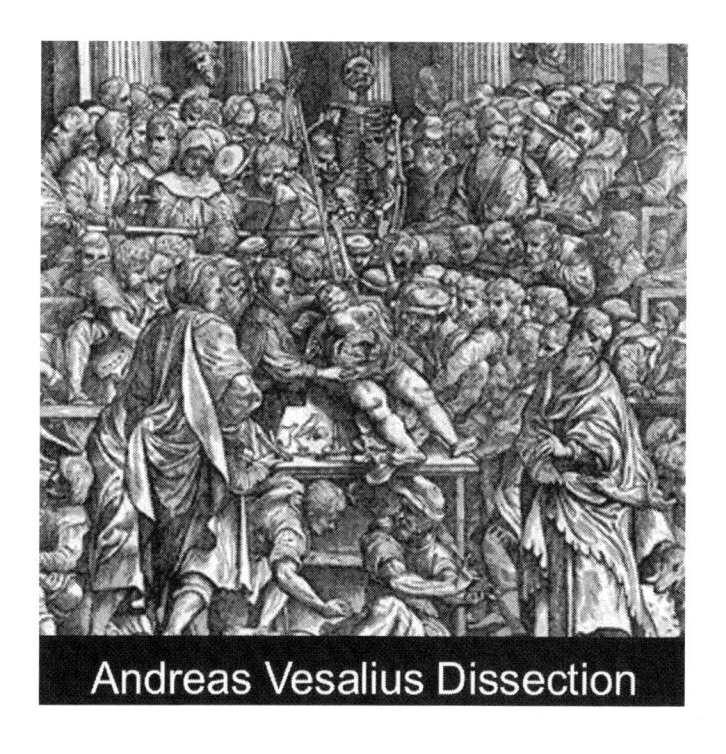

Andreas Vesalius (1514-1564), the brilliant anatomist, performed dissections and published his famous *De corporis humani fabrica* (*On the Fabric of the Human Body*) which depicted the first accurate drawings of human anatomy. His work dramatically advanced the medical arts.

The prohibition of human dissection represented a low point in medical history, but we may actually be in a worse position today. Four centuries during the Dark Ages may seem like a long time, but not in "science-time" as opposed to ordinary time. Science-time measures time as it relates to available knowledge and technology.

After all, in the 12$^{th}$ Century, there were few books, and no tissue cultures, microscopes or imaging devices like MRI machines. The most important information took years to disseminate, translate and study by the educated elite. Research based on international collaboration was unheard of. A *century* of science-time in the past may equal a *month* of science-time in the present.

## Embryonic Stem Cells

Embryonic Stem Cells (ES Cells) are derived from early stage embryos four or five days after fertilization which are comprised of 50-150 cells. These cells are nothing short of miraculous. ES Cells are pluripotent, which means they can transform into any of the other 220 types of human cells.

ES Cell therapies have been proposed for tissue replacement after age-related degeneration, traumatic injury or disease. Potentially, any number of diseases could be treated by pluripotent stem cells, including a number of genetic diseases, cancers, juvenile diabetes, Parkinson's, Alzheimer's, blindness and spinal cord injuries.

Awesome? Absolutely -- if we were allowed to perform ES Cell research without limits. But we aren't.

In 1995, Congress banned use of federal funds "for the creation of a human embryo or embryos for research purposes" or for "research in which a human embryo or embryos are destroyed, discarded, or knowingly subjected to risk of injury or death."

At the time, there were twenty-one viable embryonic stem cell lines in existence. The ban on creating new ES Cell lines for research continues to this day, although in 2009, federal funding was restored for research on existing lines created before 2001, and on lines created in private laboratories.

Thus, ES Cell research continues, but is severely hobbled by laws which prohibit creating new cell lines to study with federal research dollars. At issue are ethical questions about destroying embryos only four days old. The truth is we should be throwing money at ES Cell research. Congressmen whose last venture into the scientific arena was their 9$^{th}$ grade Earth Science class seem bound and determined to thwart one of our greatest potential leaps into the future of medicine.

The bright side is this: because government funding for new cell lines is off the table, the opportunity to invest in ES Cell research is ripe. (Pace: Mr. McGuire) There's a great future in ES Cells. Ask anyone at Geron Corporation.

Likewise on the bright side there is ongoing research in cells we all produce called the Adult Stem Cell (AS Cell). These cells vary in their potential for transformation into different cell types, and replace dying cells and regenerate damaged organs. Most importantly, they have the ability to divide or self-renew indefinitely.

AS Cells are not nearly as plastic as ES Cells, but thankfully, they are not under the thumb of scientifically challenged legislators. To date, there have been about 1,600 fascinating studies on AS Cells, and the results are promising. There have been no complete studies on ES Cells; not one.

Adult stem cells are also fairly easy to harvest and bank. While they may be useful only to the actual donor or a closely related DNA match, they can be stored indefinitely. Hopefully, the science of growing organs from AS Cells will surge forward in our lifetimes. Plan on banking your AS Cells. Twenty years from now, you may need a new heart or lung, and by then, it just might be possible to grow one in laboratory from your banked AS Cells.

## Telomeres and Anti-Telomerase

In order for any cell to divide, the complete DNA content of the cell must replicate. The two strands of the DNA molecule separate, and then the missing halves are copied.

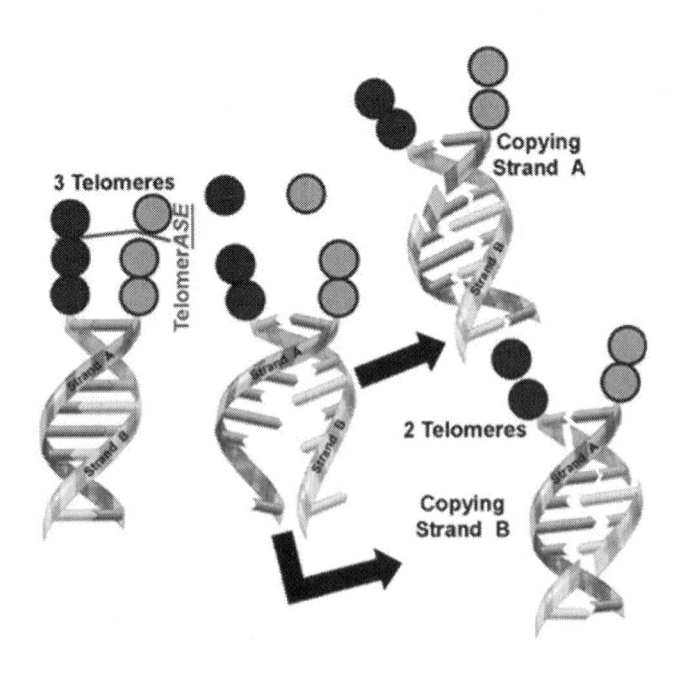

In the above illustration, we see that each strand of DNA had three end pieces represented as balls. These end pieces are called Telomeres. Every time a DNA strand divides and copies itself, it loses one of these Telomeres. This happens because of the activity of an enzyme called Telomerase.

When the DNA in a particular cell has no more Telomeres, it can no longer divide and it dies. If, however, we can prevent Telomerase from cutting off a Telomere, that cell can keep dividing and replicating its DNA with virtually no end in sight. In other words, immortal cells -- a very cool idea! The substance we're looking for would be called Anti-Telomerase.

Cancer cells seem to have an as-of-yet unidentified natural anti-telomerase. In fact, cancer cell lines are pretty much immortal, which is one of the reason cancers are so hard to kill. If we find a way to block cancer's natural anti-telomerase, we might be able to stop cancer cells from dividing. In other words, we could cure cancer.

**Anti-Aging Physicians**
The future of Anti-Aging Medicine is in the hands of individual practitioners committed to its advancement. Our calling and most important job is to change the stodgy, out-dated paradigm of traditional medicine. The time to infuse modern patient care with the promise of continued wellness is overdue. We must move beyond simply treating recurrent bouts of disease.

As science and technology advance, physicians must transition from being healers of the sick to becoming facilitators for the healthy. That transformation is long overdue.

Made in the USA
Lexington, KY
17 August 2012